CASES IN MALADJUSTMENT

CASES IN MALADJUSTMENT

The Desperate Search

Richard T. MacDougal

Dean Junior College

HarperCollins*Publishers*

Acquisitions Editor: Catherine Woods
Project Editor: Thomas R. Farrell
Cover Design: Stacey Agin
Production Manager/Assistant: Willie Lane/Sunaina Sehwani
Compositor: Ampersand
Printer and Binder: R. R. Donnelley & Sons Company
Cover Printer: New England Book Components, Inc.

Cases in Maladjustment: The Desperate Search

Library of Congress Cataloging-in-Publication Data

MacDougal, Richard T.
  Cases in maladjustment : the desperate search / Richard T.
  MacDougal.
     p.   cm/.
  Includes bibliographical references (p.   ).
  ISBN 0-673-46400-8
  1. Psychology, Pathological—Case studies. 2. Psychiatry—Case
studies.   I. Title.
  RC465.M26 1992
  616.89—dc20   91-41647
                                           CIP

92 93 94 95 9 8 7 6 5 4 3 2 1

Contents

Preface ix

Chapter 1
What Is Normal? 1
    Jerry F.: Jerry Is Cool. Jerry Is Normal
    Introduction 1
    The Case of Jerry F. 1
    Questions for Discussion 6

Chapter 2
Life Stress 7
    Temporary Situational Stress Overload
    Christy M.: I Think I Can, I Think I Can
    Introduction 7
    The Case of Christy M. 9
    Questions for Discussion 14

Chapter 3
Overdefensiveness 15
    The Best Defense Is a Stinging Offense
    Sarah J.: Winning Is the *Only* Thing
    Introduction 15
    The Case of Sarah J. 16
    Questions for Discussion 20

Chapter 4
The Escape and Avoid Choice 21
    Bill O.: I'm Very Happy Here in My Room
    Introduction 21
    The Saga of Suzie and Bill 23
    Questions for Discussion 26

Chapter 5
Phobia   27
A Symbolic Escape
Maria D.: The Fangs of Guilt
Introduction   27
Common Features of Phobias   29
The Case of Maria D.   31
Questions for Discussion   33

Chapter 6
Hysteria   35
Adjustment Through Disability (I'm Too Sick to Meet the Test Today)
Nancy L.: You Have to Consider My Condition
Introduction   35
The Case of Nancy L.   38
Questions for Discussion   40

Chapter 7
Alcohol Abuse   41
A Chemical Escape
Mike S.: Happiness Is Being Numb
Introduction   41
The Case of Mike S.   45
Questions for Discussion   51

Chapter 8
Other Substance Abuse: Cocaine   53
What Goes Up Must Come Down, Down, Down
John E.: How High This Guy
Introduction   53
The Case of John E.   57
Questions for Discussion   65

Chapter 9
Eating Disorder: Anorexia   67
The Deadly Diet
June S.: "You Can't Be Too Thin"
Introduction   67
The Case of June S.   70
Questions for Discussion   74

Chapter 10
Eating Disorder: Bulimia   75
    What Goes Down Must Come Up
    Amy O.: Purge the Contamination
    Introduction 75
    The Syndrome 76
    The Case of Amy O. 81
    Questions for Discussion 88

Chapter 11
Gender-Identity Adjustment: Homosexuality   89
    The So-called "Insult to Nature"
    Roberto V.: Why Am I Different?
    Introduction 89
    The Case of Roberto V. 93
    Questions for Discussion 98
    Bibliography 98

Chapter 12
Depression   101
    The Common Cold of Mental Illness
    Emily D.: What's the Point of Going On?
    Introduction 101
    Definitions and Forms 101
    Causes 103
    Symptoms and Characteristics 103
    How to Counteract Depression 104
    The Case of Emily D. 106
    Questions for Discussion 110

Appendix: Some Important Terms and Concepts   111

Preface

TO THE INSTRUCTOR

To paraphrase an old saying, "Necessity is the mother of creativity."

Over the past 25 years, I have learned to say to my psychology of adjustment classes every other week or so, "Let's take a break from my lectures and your test preparations. We need to take some time to have a good probing discussion of a typical case that illustrates what we have been talking about lately." Then I assign them a case to read and think about before our next class, usually two days hence.

In the early days it was relatively easy to find anthologies of case studies suitable for this kind of assignment. However, in the last several years the task has become more difficult. In spite of its tendency to stay loyal to some theoretical models of psychopathology for too long, the science of clinical psychology does move and change and challenge itself, albeit slowly. The most recent changes have been somewhat dictated, in the last decade or two, by continuing research into the complexities of how the human brain works. Discoveries in this area have brought us to entirely new models for understanding schizophrenia, homosexuality, alcoholism, and manic depression, for example. In fact, we now must consider the role of brain chemistry in virtually all psychopathologies, including neuroses such as phobias and obsessive compulsions.

As a result of this research, the old anthologies were becoming outdated and inaccurate and, as far as I could determine, no satisfactory new ones were being published. The only solution, it seemed, was to write my own.

In putting these cases together in book form, I assumed that there are other professors out there with similar needs who are trying to teach the psychology of adjustment, and similar life-related courses, to relatively inexperienced students of psychology. With this in mind, I attempted to keep the discussions from becoming too technically sophisticated. On the other hand, it is important that the student come to achieve some literacy in the language of psychology, so I have tried to achieve a balance. I have also tried to select interesting stories that can be read in one sitting. This book is intended to be a supplementary text, not a principal textbook. However, because it is a teaching aid, the coordinating explanations attempt to help the student to understand the psychodynamics of each variety of maladjustment.

Therefore, I include a list of directive questions, which students refresh in their minds before reading each case. Some of the questions can provide the basis for discussion of the case in class—or at least can get it started. I advise them to keep the list in their case books—perhaps to use as a bookmark, which keeps it handy.

While other instructors may want to use additional questions, more consistent with their own theoretical orientation, I submit the following as the general questions that can be used with the cases. More questions are included, specific to the individual case, after each case story.

Questions for Study, Discussion, and Understanding

1. What is the behavior in question "saying"? What can we infer or hypothesize regarding the individual's important underlying motives and needs?
2. What is the predominant kind of adjustment pattern that the individual seems to have chosen? For example, does he or she tend to attack or run away from threat?
3. How does the individual perceive, in general, the world? Is it comfortable, ambiguous, or threatening? How does this perception correlate with the person's dominant feelings?
4. What is the nature of the individual's self-concept? Typically, how high or low is the level of self-esteem? Is it constant and consistent or variable? What kinds of words would be used to complete the phrase: I am _____?
5. How integrative/nonintegrative are the predominant adjustment patterns? (Please see the explanation of these terms in the Appendix.)
6. How well prepared or trained is the individual to make healthy adjustments to difficulties or stress? How adequate are his or her psychological resources? To what extent are they limited? Why?

Note that none of the above questions asks the student to diagnose a problem in terms of labeling categories, such as according to psychiatry's *DSM IIIR*. I make every effort to avoid the use of diagnostic labels with introductory students. This kind of labeling is unnecessarily technical; it is unreliable, vague, inconsistent, and subjective; and too often it is misleading or inaccurate, and perpetuates the common social error of tagging people with labels from which they may never successfully free themselves. I prefer to teach a more useful system, which focuses on kinds of adjustive *behavior* (in the manner of Karen Horney, for example), and allows for the perception of the possibility of change and growth. Even the terms neurosis and psychosis are useful only to convey the idea of relative degrees of maladjustment along a continuum from moderate to severe.

Note also that neither the selection of the case example nor the explanation presupposes any particular theoretical orientation or bias. In fact, I tend to discourage this. While beginning students of clinical psychology need to be thoroughly exposed to psychoanalytic, behavioristic, and humanistic theory and language (at the very least from an historical perspective), they should not become engaged, let alone married, to any one theory too early in their education. In fact, I encourage eclecticism, if this implies flexibility, acknowledgment of new research, and the awareness that seldom does a case adapt itself perfectly to a single theoretical system of diagnosis and treatment. If I lean in any particular direction, it is toward a learning model. I believe it is easiest for beginning students to learn to apply to everyday problems the idea that one can learn maladjustive habits just as easily as more healthy ones. I emphasize the critical role of the self-concept in determining the quality of one's adjustment to everyday situations. I also teach a humble awareness of the imperfections of our science, and that we must continue to keep an open mind and some curiosity about the progress of psychobiology toward understanding the role of brain chemistry in maladaptive thinking.

TO THE STUDENT

In my classes I try to make each course educationally valid as well as life useful, regardless of why the student registered for the course in the first place. I believe this should be a goal of all psychology courses. While some students may never take another course in psychology, others will go on to major in it or even become counselors or therapists. No matter what path one chooses toward a productive and happy life, it is a necessity to acquire the ability and desire to interact effectively with other human beings. This involves many skills, which our culture attempts to teach us from childhood on. Foremost among these skills is the ability to understand other people's needs and feelings, as well as one's own. This is a major goal of the analysis and discussion of a case study. It involves continually asking the question, "What is this behavior saying or suggesting to us about the person's needs and feelings?" If "all behavior is motivated," then we are aided measurably by this approach in gaining insight into "where a person is coming from." It is essential in effective communication, especially between intimates, but it also represents a giant step forward toward insight into even some of the most bizarre behavior.

The reading of a case study by a student is part of a course of study. It therefore should be purposeful. Although I have attempted to make the cases interesting, a case study should not be read as if it were canned fantasy or recreational literature. It is part of the educational process. Since education is the search for answers to questions, then you should read a case study in the same purposeful manner as text reading—looking for answers to questions.

ACKNOWLEDGMENTS

Becoming a writing teacher after years of being a talking teacher turned out to be a more complicated process than I anticipated. And it required the help of many people. Although my overwhelming memory of the book-writing process is of the hundreds of hours of solitary labor, the truth is, a book doesn't get published without the assistance of other people, in smaller but very important ways. There are those who let me use their stories, whose identities I hope I have carefully protected. There are my devoted readers, who have been so generous with their time and constructive criticism. And there are the editors who believed in my project. To all of the following people (listed in no particular order), and more, I give my sincere appreciation: Toni M., Stephanie C., Cheryl B., John, Julie D., Tom P., Ardyth E., Dottie G., Sidney M., Ed H., Sarah M., Charlie J., Bob H., Jeff J., Don H., Marge J., Ann H., Debby H., and of course, Betsy M. I also acknowledge the invaluable contributions of the critical reviewers:

Barbara J. Hermann, Gainesville College
Joan Rosen, Miami-Dade Community College
David L. Andrews, Indiana State University
Charles G. Frederickson, Centenary College
Jerry Walke, Shawnee State University
Mary Kenning, University of Nebraska at Lincoln
Paul Frick, University of Alabama
Thomas J. Schoeneman, Lewis and Clark University

RICHARD T. MACDOUGAL

Chapter
1

What Is Normal?

JERRY F: JERRY IS COOL. JERRY IS NORMAL

Introduction: Am I Crazy? Am I OK? Am I Normal?

In the vernacular, or common language, every day people struggle to find the right words to express an idea or a questions about being well or badly adjusted. To illustrate this point, I have on occasion asked my classes to repeat all the words they have heard to mean mentally disturbed, while I listed their contributions on the chalkboard. A typical list includes crazy, insane, screwy, bonkers, round the bend, flaky, out of it, abnormal. It is obvious that it is a difficult concept to pin down.

Even more frustrating is the attempt to find a satisfactory vocabulary to convey the opposite meaning—a healthy or well-adjusted personality. It is somewhat reassuring to the students when I call their attention to one of their first assignments in the textbook. It explains that, historically, well-known theorists and authors have had just as much difficulty agreeing on the most effective language to convey this idea of well or poorly adjusted, and what the criteria should be. To make matters worse, I usually disagree with some terminology and points of view in our textbook. Consistently, one of the most popular words used is "normal." It seems to be the most common antonym for words meaning "a little crazy." I hear it used almost every day. "Am I normal?"; "She's so normal"; "You're the most normal person I know, nothing seems to bother you." "Normal" seems to be the most convenient word to convey the idea of well adjusted. But how accurate is it? Consider the case of Jerry F.

The Case of Jerry F.

Jerry gave people a first impression of being a very normal student on our campus, or any other. He was a little above average in height, well-

1

proportioned, athletic looking, and was probably considered handsome by his mother and his female peers. With the other guys, he was typical. He shuffled around campus in untied high-top sneakers, jeans, and a well-worn sweatshirt with frayed cut-off sleeves. His blonde hair was right in style that year— shaved up the sides, with a considerable length hanging down the back of his neck.

Jerry had an easy, unruffled social style; he easily made witty conversation and jokes using all the current jargon and slang. He knew all the popular tunes and rock groups; and was almost always found in a cluster of his male and female friends, who shared similar interests and style. Jerry was cool. Jerry was normal.

In the middle of the first semester, on the Saturday when parents were invited to visit the campus and meet with faculty, Jerry's parents dutifully accepted the invitation and conscientiously waited in line in order to have a talk with all five of Jerry's professors. When their turn came at my office, I found myself shaking hands warmly with an attractive, well-dressed, socially graceful, middle-aged couple. In order to take Jerry to dinner, they had driven up the night before from their home in an affluent community in southern Connecticut, where Mr. F. owned his own successful business. After the initial social amenities, the conversation became much more businesslike. I suddenly became aware of my using subtle defensive strategies to sidestep their questions regarding how I was going to help Jerry improve his performance. He had received a D− on the first test, and his parents wondered if I could arrange for special tutorial help.

It seems that the original plan was for Jerry to attend Yale, Mr. F.'s alma mater. This plan had to be postponed in favor of enrollment in a junior college, as a result of Jerry's interest in social activities and sports, which had jeopardized his academic standing. He barely graduated from high school, and his grades would not even get him into the state college.

Jerry's parents' goals for Jerry included a successful career in the family business, after he received bachelor's and master's degrees in business. Jerry identified with these goals, or at least paid them lip service, and registered as a business major at the junior college.

When I deflected to Jerry his parents' questions about "getting him back on the track," and what *he* was going to do about the problem, he mumbled something vague like, "work harder, I guess." My intuitive reaction was that he had no idea what that meant, but it sounded good, and would appease the people paying the bill—at least for now. In the few minutes remaining, I outlined a program of improved attendance, work habits, and test preparation, designed to get him "back on the track" by the end of the semester, at least in my course. Jerry listened obediently and with a visible sense of relief that someone was responding satisfactorily to his parents' questions.

As they left the office, I could read clearly in Jerry's demeanor how relieved he would be when this ordeal of the duty tour of faculty conferences was over. I had many similar conferences that day; Jerry's case was very "normal."

It was not until several months later that I became aware of the enormity of the nonintegrativeness° of Jerry's seemingly "normal" behavior and lifestyle. At the time, all I knew was that Jerry had earned his D− in my psychology course. He had three times the allowed number of absences, had done very superficial reading of his textbook, and written an almost incomprehensible essay on the first test. In class, he was one of those students who has developed skills for being unnoticed in the back of the room whenever the teacher throws a direct question to the class—much like the rabbit that instinctively remains motionless in the presence of danger. His infrequent contributions to class discussion consisted of witty remarks, well designed to attract approving attention from his peers, but totally unrelated to the question.

His performance in other courses was even worse. He had slept through roughly half of his 8:00 A.M. classes, as a result of partying the night before, or simply through a lack of self-discipline. He had cut about the same number of Friday classes, choosing instead to take off early for party weekends off campus. He was passing—barely—his freshman English composition course, solely because it commenced with a remedial review that reached back to the pre-junior high school level of his skills. Although he communicated easily with his peers, his lack of commitment to academic pursuits had caused him to finish the first 12 years of school with a primitive, almost nonexistent knowledge of the formal English language. He had no comprehension of proper sentence structure or rules of grammar, his spelling was an immature approximation of sound, and his vocabulary was so limited that the semantics of any textbook left him bewildered.

Unfortunately, Jerry's very normal pursuit of today's satisfactions, without regard for tomorrow's consequences, produced the almost inevitable result. After being on academic warning for the spring semester, he was withdrawn from the college in June for an unacceptably low grade point average, with the provision that if he achieved grades of C or better in two summer courses, he would be readmitted for the fall semester, on academic probation.

He somehow managed to meet this requirement with two easy courses taken at a state community college near his parents' summer home at the shore. With his own car he easily made the daily morning commute during June and July. He had most of his afternoons free to "cruise the beach for chicks" and the month of August to perfect his tan.

By the middle of the next fall semester, his probationary status with the academic dean was more than matched by his standing with the dean of student affairs—with whom he was in double trouble. He had been issued the final warning after this third violation of the campus alcohol regulations, and for harrassment of a female student and willful destruction of college property. I became involved in the case at this point, when Jerry requested counseling sessions with me in lieu of mandatory appointments at the college counseling center, which were part of his disciplinary probation requirements.

°For a thorough discussion of the important terms *integrative* and *nonintegrative,* refer to the Appendix.

Although he had not learned much psychology in my class the previous year, he said he had "enjoyed" some of the classes and felt he would be more comfortable talking with me that with an unknown person at the counseling center. The dean agreed to this request because of my expertise in the area of alcohol abuse problems.

The Jerry F. who arrived at my office was a very different person from the "cool" sophomore seen by most of the rest of the campus. He showed extensive signs of stress. He was agitated, hyperactive, tired looking, and anxious—frequently drying his sweaty hands on the sides of his jeans. His usual practiced casual appearance had become disheveled and careless. He immediately began to talk in a desperate, nonstop flow of disconnected thoughts, which had built up for some time. And the intensity of his concerns had become magnified by his anxiety preceding his talk with the "shrink." Jerry had lost his "cool." Worse, he had lost control—of his life, his future, his freedom of choice, and, worst of all, of his own impulses.

For a while, I allowed him the catharsis of talking, but eventually had to step in to calm him and put him at ease, so that we could begin to organize his problems with some directive questions. The situation that resulted in this personal crisis and the last-straw ultimatum from the dean was not really so complicated. His on-campus girl friend had finally tired of his drinking, his immature selfishness, and the limited, physical basis of the relationship, and had taken up company with another young man. Jerry's unsuccessful attempts to badger her into changing her mind culminated in a drunken, jealous rage during which he scratched obscenities into the door of her dorm room and screamed vulgar names and threats at her through the door. When driven from the dormitory by a residence director, he threw a rock through the window of her room, wrapped in an obscene note. This was followed by a bloody fist fight with his rival, who had interceded to protect the girl friend.

Counseling a young adult who is functioning on the level of a spoiled child throwing a temper tantrum is a difficult process. During our second session I sensed that Jerry was going to resume his irresponsible course of action if we did not begin to make more progress in counseling and keep him from digging himself even deeper into his hole. Consequently, I adopted a more short-term, directive approach. First I pointed out that to continue his defensive, blame-seeking railing against that "fickle bitch," and the "f___king, narrow-minded, vindictive dean" would be pointless and regressive. I refused to waste time listening to any more of it. Second, it would be helpful if he could refocus his attention away from his obsessive preoccupation with his sexual needs. Third, I insisted that he reduce drastically the amount of time his brain was having to function in an alcohol bath. It simply cannot function normally in that environment. I also stated that I would no longer counsel him unless he has been sober for 24 hours prior to a session, that my time was too valuable to waste trying to cope with a mind rendered incapable of learning anything. Fourth, I insisted on seeing real effort being made to wrest control from the hedonistic, spoiled child who had been governing his daily activities and decisions for too long. Only after he began to meet these requirements

could I begin to help him to focus on longer-range goals, needs, and consequences, and to make some progress toward maturity and adulthood. He had
to realize that these should be a top priority at his age. Actually, he needed little reminding, because part of his anger was due to the awareness of how immature the intensity of his jealousy had been. And, from this point, it was surprisingly easy to get him to see the correlation between his irresponsibility
and partying (and particularly his drinking) and the rest of his problems.

Jerry managed somewhat to "clean up his act," and stay out of further
trouble with the student affairs office for the rest of the semester. But there
was simply not enough time to improve the dismal state of his grade point
average. In addition, his improved motivation could not offset his deficient
verbal skills. The academic office issued Jerry a permanent dismissal in
December. Actually, this would not have been necessary, for, although his
parents had spoiled him for too many years, Jerry's father was a good business-
man and had already decided that there was too little return on his more than
$15,000 investment in Jerry's three semesters at a private junior college. He
shut off additional funds for this purpose.

The rest of Jerry's story is not known. We do know that when he left the
college his life and his self-esteem were a mess. Nevertheless, we have to say
that Jerry was normal relative to his peers. He was, in fact, very much like most
of his peers in many ways.

To finish our discussion, let us return to our initial question: What is normal and should we use the term to mean well adjusted? Normal is a valid term
only when used in a statistical context. It refers to frequency, and when applied to behavior means typical, most common, or average, It is always
relative—to cultural norms, at different times, to different parts of the culture,
and to what is typical for an individual. Its opposite term, abnormal, therefore
means different, atypical, nonconforming, eccentric, unconventional, or even
bizarre. None of these words, when applied to behavior, necessarily implies a
maladjusted or unhealthy personality. The ability of a person, an adolescent,
for example, *not* to conform to a nonintegrative norm may indicate a stronger,
healthier personality—with possibly a much better prognosis for becoming a
well-adjusted, fulfilled adult.

So Let us try to avoid the temptation to use "normal" to mean well adjusted or healthy, from a psychological point of view. Our communication will be
much improved for the effort.

There is a last important point to keep in mind. All psychopathology, no
matter how bizarre, is only an exaggeration of the normal realistic functioning
of the mind. Everyone uses defense mechanisms. Everyone has fears that are
somewhat unreasonable. And everyone is capable of illogical flights of
fantasy—we have only to recall our most recent "weird" dream to appreciate this.

In the same manner, mental aberrations caused by imbalances of brain
biochemistry (and modern medical science is coming to include more and
more psychopathologies in this category) can be the result of a tiny amount of

variation in the normal amount of a brain neurotransmitter that is at work. Thus, "normal" actually includes a fairly wide range in the middle of a continuum of human mental functioning.

QUESTIONS FOR DISCUSSION

1. Relative to your experience and your peer group, do you think Jerry was normal?
2. Do you think Jerry was well adjusted? Was he more or less so at different times?
3. As indicators of his self-concept, what kind of words do you think Jerry would have used to describe himself during that winter, after he was expelled from college?
4. What do you think Jerry will be like when he is 23 or 24 years old, in terms of his life-style and psychological condition?
5. Do you think any of the other important people in Jerry's life might have been able to influence changes in his behavior in a more positive direction sooner? Who would they have been? What might they have tried to do or say?
6. After reading this brief case history, would you describe your behavior and life-style as "normal"? Why do you think so? Or why not?

Chapter
2

Life Stress
Temporary Situational
Stress Overload

CHRISTY M.: I THINK I CAN, I THINK I CAN

Introduction

Human psychology is inclined to use such terms and concepts as growth, becoming, self-esteem, and self-actualization when describing human needs and motives. One of the best known and clearly described humanistic theories is Mazlow's hierarchy of human needs, conceptualized as a pyramid of layers. The foundation or bottom layer consists of basic survival needs, such as hunger, thirst, and so forth. We all must tend to these first. At the top of the stratification we move from purely physiological drives to purely psychological needs. The highest of these is called "self-actualization." The assumption is that, whether we are consciously aware of it or not, we engage in a lifelong striving to become all that we are capable of becoming, and to relize to the fullest our aptitudes and potentials. Adjustment at this level of functioning, according to Mazlow, is rate, at least on any continuing basis. And it is virtually inconceivalbe for the millions of very poor for whom life is a continuing struggle just to stay alive. For those of us who are fortunate enough to have our basic needs satisfied to the extent that we are free to pursue higher education, it is still a rare event to be working at a self-actualizing level. The reason is that we must adjust to formidable obstacles at lower levels of needs on the hierarchy. It is with these middle levels that this chapter will be concerned.

Between basic survival needs and self-actualization is the need to be loved and to learn to love, for status and social acceptance, for positive self-definition or self-esteem, and for "success" or achievement. Notice that all of these needs involve interaction with other people. Beginning with the long period of dependency of the human infant, we acquire powerful needs involving effective interaction with other people. In the beginning we could not survive physically without their care. Later, we cannot survive psychologically without their approval. "They" define what a "good person" is. And they say you must be a good person, as they define it, or they won't love you, or accept you, or let you be in their group. This "good person" eventually has many parts or roles: good son or daughter, student, friend, mother, father, employee, citizen, producer, achiever, group member.

The essential ingredient in any healthy personality is a general sense of good feelings aobut oneself. I am liked, accepted, attractive, successful, and so forth. I feel good about me. I'm OK. Because other people provide most of the input necessary for these good feelings, they exert tremendous influence or pressure on our behavior. This pressure can result in a great deal of stress, especially when different groups make conflicting demans, or when we have internalized social standards to such a degree that we pressure ourselves toward idealized, unrealistic levels of performance.

We are likely to experience some frustration in meeting all of these external and internal demands, and this frustration we experience as stress. In this case stress takes the form of anxiety or guilt from failing to meet, or fear that we won't meet, the requirements of being a "good" person. Feelings of failure or inferiority are very stressful.

Another form or source of stress—as studied in great detail by Homles et al.—is a change in accustomed life routines. it may be moving to a new residence, a new school, a new job, a new group of people. Or it may be the loss of an important intimate person in one's life—mate, parent, sibling, friend. Whatever it is, change equals stress.

It would be helpful if the stress-causing problems in our lives would come along one at a time. (It is too much to hope that there wouldn't be any.) But, alas, they tend to come in bunches. These times of problem/stress bunch-up are a good measure of one's adjustive capabilities and strength of character and personality.

The human species, like all others, has a strong motive for survival. Though life seems to throw into our paths a great variety of obstacles, problems, illnesses, and competition for our survival needs, most of us tend to muddle through and keep going. But not all of us. As we push forward on the road of life, we notice the trail of bodies by the wayside. These are people who, one by one, reached the limits of their ability to cope or endure, and collapsed or gave up. Each of us has such a limit or threshold, and for each of us it is different. Among people there is a broad continuum of ability to cope with stress. At the low end of this continuum are the few who, at the least possibility of threat or pain or difficult, just lie down saying, "I can't," "I don't know how," or "I'm too weak." We all know one or two of these people. They did not learn anything from the first-grade story of "The Little Engine That Could." "I think I can" is not in their vocabulary. At the other end of the continuum are some who, in the best tradition of the culture's ideals, continue to perservere alone, with "stiff upper lip" and "shoulder to the wheel" and "never say die," for far too long a time—long after reasonable people would have sought help or found a way to lighten the load. If one does not heed the warnings of body or mind that one has crossed the threshold or has been in the danger zone of stress-load for too long, then either or both will take their own relief by breaking down. Consider the following case.

The Case of Christy M.

In the quiet solitude of her dormitory room, Christy sat staring at an open, but scarcely tended to, history book. Just before 3:00 A.M., the dorm had finally become quiet. No longer did the stereos blare or the sounds of laughing echo down the hallways. It was time to hope for some uninterrupted study. But Christy felt too overwhelmed by fatigue and despair to focus on any more studying. What did it really matter anyway? What was the use? She desperately longed to just fold into her bed and sleep forever. How many days had it been since she had had more than two hours of sleep? But even sleep was frightening. Twice this week, when she had finally gone to sleep, early in the morning, she had had the same terrifying dream. She was walking purposefully down a dark and lonely road; there were no signs of any hourses or safe havens, or even any indication of where the road was going. She sensed danger in the darkenss but saw nothing except the eyes she imagined among the trees. Soon she was aware that a huge, slimy monster was approaching slowly on the road behind her. It had several heads, each of which had a gaping maw with rows of sharp teeth. Any one of them could have engulfed and swallowed her. Terrified, she tried to run, but each of her legs felt encased in 100 pounds of cement, so that she could barely move one in front of the other. She picked up a stick to hit the thing in self-defense, but the stick turned into a limp bunch of grass. At this point she wakened, screaming in terror. Why was life so difficult? Did it ever let up? Did it ever become easier?

Christy, at 18, was the second eldest of five children. Her older brother, Phillip, was a senior at Harvard, cruising to the end of a very successful college experience as a dean's list student and star athlete. This had followed a similar "hero" career in high school, where he was an all-state baseball player and had earned several large academic scholarships to go to Harvard. He was the apple of his father's eye—appropriate, since he was Phillip M., Jr. The three younger children included a sister in grade 11 and brothers in grades 9 and 5. They were managing to do above average schoolwork with a normal amount of effort, and were socially well adjusted within their circles of friends.

Christy often wondered to herself, "How did I get left out?" She too had wanted badly to go to a "good" college—in fact, Smith and Barnard were her dreams. This would really have pleased her parents. Mr. M. had a master's degree in education and was a school administrator in their middle-class suburb of Boston. He was the authority in the family and expected high standards of achievement. He was fair and understanding, but was not blessed with a great deal of empathy or sensitivity. Mrs. M. was an intelligent, educated woman, though quiet and unassertive. She did not work outside of the home.

Christy was a conscientious and responsible girl who never had to be badgered to help with home chores or to care for the younger children. Through high school she managed to keep most of her grades at the C− level, but only by plodding through long, dilligent hours of homework—plus extra credit work whenever it was suggested. She passed tests by sheer memorization, but seldom really understood the material to any depth. She almost never could handle a question that asked her to apply a fact or principle to a new situation. She had once had a brief testing session for the possiblity of a learning disability, but the results were inconclusive. She tried out for basketball and field hockey, but got little playing time or "hero" opportunities in either sport. Out of her hearing, the coaches referred to her as a "klutz." And though she was a pleasant, likable girl, she had only a few close friends and almost no social life. There was always too much homework to do. Whenever she wasn't needed at home by her mother, she worked many evenings at baby-sitting to "save money for college."

In Christy's senior year of high school the additions to her lists of disappointments became longer. A guidance counselor convinced her to let go of her dream of going to Smith, that it was totally unrealistic. About the time that she had rationalized the "wisdom" (especially economically) of going to a state college, she received the results of her SAT tests. Her scores were so low that she would be placed only near the bottom of the waiting list for any of the state colleges.

But the system provides a *repechage,* a second chance for losers to get back into the competition. Christy enrolled in a junior college with an open-door enrollment policy. At least she was in college, and the path to her goals was still open. In the fall she attacked the challenge of a first semester at college with her enthusiasm and determination restored by the excitment of her brother Phil's graduation ceremony and a summer's rest.

College life was not at all what christy expected. CHALLENGE now was spelled with capital letters. The stack of thick books seemed immense, and the homework began immediately. Even as conscientious as she was, she almost immediately fell behind in most of her subjects. Her curriculum included a science course for which she was poorly prepared and had no aptitude. She had had no grammatical instruction since the sixth grade, but her professors expected proper English grammar and spelling. Further, the level of understanding and application that was required made her memorizing habits even less adequate than they had been in high school. The length of the reading assignments seemed insurmountable. By the end of the first semester she was on academic probation.

Adjustment to college social life was equally difficult. Accustomed to her

---

Repechage is an Olympic Games tradition in some sports whereby losers of trial heats can compete to get back into the competition for prizes.

own private room, she now found herself with two roommates with whom she was poorly matched. Though pleasant and sociable, both of the other girls considered "partying" their first priority. Christy had no preparation for coping with the blaring stereos, cigarette smoke and frequent presense of boys in the room. She found it particularly uncomfortable to be made to feel that she had to "go somewhere" whenever one of her roommates wanted privacy with her boyfriend. Weekends presented mixed feelings. While she had the room to herself when her roommates took off for the weekend, she also envied their unlimited budgets and freedom to go home whenever they wanted. She was very homesick.

She was also very tired. Working two jobs, one an on-campus student "workship" and the other an off-campus job at a fast food restaurant, cut down on the time needed for study. Sleep was always a precious commodity. However, she somehow managed to survive the second semester with a reduced course load and some tutoring assistance. But she was still on probation, and finishing the two-year curriculum was a big question mark. She seemed never to feel free of the awful pressure.

Halfway through her third semester, fate curelly added more burdens to her stress load. At home during a long holiday weekend, she learned that her younger sister, Jean, was in trouble. With Christy and her stabilizing influence away at school, Jean had joined a more adventurous group of friends and had recently discovered that she was pregnant. Christy worried frequently about the difficult decisions to be made and the possible effects on Jean's life. Then, in early November, her mother called to tell her that Mr. M. had suffered a serious heart attack. He would be out of work for several months, and there was serious concern that there would be a second and fatal attack. This was the kind of worry about which one feels totally helpless. It also meant that, even though her third semester was paid for, there would be no money for a fourth semester.

In the middle of November, with genuine sympathy, Christy's roommates prevailed on her to "lighten up" and accompany them to a party. After a couple of mixed drinks, which were a little stronger than they tasted, she actually began to have a good time, thanks also to a young man named Jim who took an interest in her and spent most of the evening with her. Shortly thereafter she entered into her first meaningful sexual relationship. She was flattered by his desire to spend all of his spare time with her and was comforted for a time by the physical intimacy.

But shortly thereafter she broke off with Jim, realizing that his interest was primarily physical rather than leading to a complete relationship. The affair was also cutting into her study time. She was alone again.

Next she had to face a history test. Shortly after mid-semester she had received a warning letter from the academic office reminding her that if she did not meet the minimum GPA requirement by the end of the semester, she would be withdrawn from the college for academic failure. History was one of her two most difficult courses because of the amount of required reading. She was failing the course at this point, so this test was critical. If she did not pass it, there would be no point in even taking the final exam, and it would be impossible to meet the required GPA. To exacerbate the problem, she also had an English test that week that also required much reading. Preparation for the history test was exhausting. She spent many hours, including two all-night sessions, plodding through material that was of little interest to her. As she walked into the Friday morning test, she was spent, barely running on fumes. There was nothing left. Her head felt as though full of wet sand and her eyes would barely focus. Afterward, she really did not know if she had passed the test or not.

Christy sat with great anxiety in class waiting. At 10 past the hour the professor came in, not with the test results but with the announcement that it had been discovered that someone had managed to steal a copy of the test from the department secretary's office. Because it was not possible to discover how many people had benefited from the theft, the exam would be repeated at the next class. This time the test would be all essays, a more difficult form for Christy. She had spent the weekend finishing an overdue psychology paper and had a bad cold and felt rotten. How could she possibly study for another history test? As she sat staring with unseeing eyes at the history book in the lonely quiet of her room, Christy's resolve ran out and her coping resources collapsed. She began to sob and wail uncontrollably.

At 7:30 the following morning, when a roommate returned to get ready for an early class, she found Christy wimpering and rocking, sitting at the head of her bed, cradled by the junction of two walls, arms wrapped tightly around her legs. No amount of urging or encouragement would elicit a response—a withdrawn child had escaped into her own sefe haven, immune from further pain.

The roommate called the resident director, who called the health service. Neither a college counselor nor the consulting psychologist was able to bring Christy very far out of her withdrawal. Her mother was called to take her home. Christy's college career was over.

We are left wondering about the prognosis for Christy's future. How long, if ever, will it be before she returns to her normal self? How has her self-concept been affected? Has she learned something useful about her own limits? Will she ever again try to take on so heavy a load? To lose control is very frightening and one is usually careful to try to prevent it from happening again.

Earlier we discussed thresholds or limits of a person's ability to cope with or endure stress. In this context it is useful to refer to the research of Hans Selye, which has made an important contribution to our understanding of human stress. You will likely study his theory in your course. Selye described human adjustment to stress in terms of a general adaptation syndrome. Diagrammed it looks something like Figure 2.1.

Three variables make the shape of the chart different for each individual:

1. The magnitude of the problem as it is perceived by the individual and the amount and kind of adjustive resources he or she has to call upon, in the alarm stage.

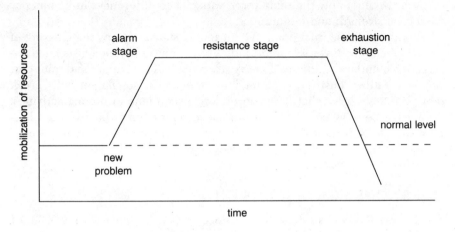

Figure 2.1 Human adjustment to stress.

2. The amount of time an individual can continue to persevere in the resistence stage, trying to cope with the problem, or to keep saying "I think I can."
3. The kind and severity of symptoms that develop in the exhaustion stage.

Of course, each additional problem calls upon the individual to muster additional coping resources, if possible.

Let us simplify the discussion by switching from the subject of psychological strength to an example of differences in physical strength. Let's say that I take 100 students, stand them in a line, and fasten large pack baskets on their backs. Next, I walk up and down the line, each time dropping a 5-pound stone in each basket. Fairly soon a first person will drop down saying, "That's all I can carry." With each pass a few more will reach their "last stone" threshold and drop out. At the end two large students will battle it out, but eventually only one will remain. There may be a difference of more than 200 pounds between the first and the last. What variables make up the wide range of difference in load-carrying capacity? I suggest that there are least three:

1. Inherent muscle mass or strength.
2. Practice, training, and conditioning—what kind of shape the person is in.
3. Attitude and motivation—how disposed the person is to keep saying, "I can do it," "I think I can."

I was fascinated as I watched the complex interaction among the variables in the weightlifting competition in the last Olympic Games. Here individuals of identical size and weight, in each body-weight class, sometimes lift weights in excess of three times their body weight over their heads. This feat is inconceivable to average normal people.

Can we not apply the same three variables to differences in human psychological strength and endurance?

I will make one final point. An intriguing statistic keeps reappearing in studies of coping. Over a long period of time clinical psychologists have observed that under conditions of heavy stress, such as the danger and trauma of war and battle, consistently about 20 percent of a population will "break down" to the degree that they can no longer continue in normal activities. They must be relieved of duty or normal responsibilities and are often hospitalized. What is the difference between these people and the 80 percent who are survivors? Is it the same three factors?

QUESTIONS FOR DISCUSSION

1. What was Christy's "last straw" (or "last stone"), when she stopped saying, "I think I can"?
2. How would you describe her self-concept? Why? How realistic were her self-perception and her expections?
3. Did she give up (go down) without a fight?
4. Why did she wind up in the 20 percent who break down?
5. How do you think she could have kept her stress load at a more manageable level?
6. Did you attempt to interpret Christy's dream? What do you think some of the details symbolize?
7. Which of the general questions from the preface are applicable in this case?
8. What are the implications from this case for better management of your own life adjustment?

Chapter
3

Overdefensiveness
The Best Defense
Is a Stinging Offense

SARAH J.: WINNING IS THE *ONLY* THING

Introduction: The Basic Choices to Deal with Threat

Whenever an individual is confronted with a situation that is perceived as threatening to his or her well-being, there is an automatic arousal in every part of the body readying him or her to deal with the danger. This is true of all animals. Although we do not speak of human instincts, this instant increase of physical and mental alertness is a fully automatic response of the autonomic nervous system. Human uniqueness comes from the great range of choices from which we can select the best to cope with the particular threat. We may fight, run away, or hide; we may just stop and think about it, try to negotiate, or find a way to pretend that there is no danger at all.

Although psychologists may not agree on how many different choices there are in the human repertoire of defense, there is fairly general agreement that these choices fall into two main types or categories: stand and fight or run away and escape. This dichotomy is referred to by many labels—Fight or flight, Offensive or Avoidance, Advance or Retreat, Moving Against or Moving Away From, but each still describes the two main options. Most people have a preferred style and we recognize it as part of their personalities. Individual preference probably results from a combination of innate predisposition and learning from successful life experiences. A healthy personality is marked by a flexibility to decide which kind of adjustment is most appropriate for a given situation. Typical of poorly adjusted people is a tendency to have little flexibility, to choose repeatedly the same adjustive behavior even if it usually makes matters worse for them in the long run. This is the point that I will illustrate below and in Chapter 4.

Let us look first at an example of a person whose personality shows a distinct preference for dealing with threat from interpersonal relations in a manner that is aggressive, offensive, and assertive. Karen Horney called this kind of social behavior "moving against people." The person will consistently choose this kind of adjustive style as if no other choices were available. The person's behavior tends to be antisocial and to increase the social distance between him or her and other people. Ironically, this result is quite the opposite result from what the person is striving for. These behaviors are well-established habits and, as you probably have observed, are difficult to change. Such adjustive habits are correctly referred to as defense mechanisms.

Keep in mind that when we speak of social threat we mean threat to self-esteem from the behavior of other people. Therefore, the purpose of these defense mechanisms is to defend or protect the self-concept. Every one of us has a defense system—a set of preferred defense mechanisms—that we have established over the years. Therefore, defense mechanisms are normal, because no one likes to be made to feel inferior or have one's "feelings hurt" by the actions or words of others.

However, you must have noticed that some people are more defensive than others. You may have found yourself referring to one of these people in this way: "She is so insecure; you have to be so careful what you say around her." These people tend to overreact, or to become defensive when threat is only a possibility or is perceived where no one else saw it or it was not intended. Negative earlier experiences have conditioned them to be wary in *any* situation that might involve comparison or evaluation or criticism. These people do not have comfortable, confident, secure, or healthy self-concepts—their world is full of possible danger. I refer to a person like this as an over-defensive person. His or her defensiveness is not "normal." When the over-defensive person chooses an assortment of "fight" mechanisms as the defensive style, the result can be a dramatic example of a maladjusted person.

Let us consider the case of Sarah J., an acquaintance of mine from some years ago. It may sound familar to you and will provide valuable insights into the dynamics of how efforts to achieve satisfactory social adjustment can go sour.

The Case of Sarah J.

Sarah was one of those students who seem to draw the focus of others' attention, almost from the moment she stepped on campus, because she worked at it. There was an intensity and "busy-ness" about her. Whatever she was doing seemed very purposeful and important. Getting acquainted was not difficult. She quickly became energetically involved in any group conversation comparing personal backgrounds and histories. Before long, most of the young women in the dorm had heard stories of the escapades, victories, and championships that she had accomplished in her high school. A number of students could recall being interrupted when telling their own stories.

She was soon well known in the Office of Student Affairs and remained so throughout most of her four years of college. By the end of her freshman year she engendered mixed feelings among the assistant deans and project advisors. While she could do a very good job at whatever she put her attention to, she seemed to be involved in too many activities. She was one of the first to run for election as the representative for her dorm in the student government. She became a member of the yearbook staff, and the student disciplinary committee, and was a reporter/photographer for the college newspaper.

She became equally well known on other parts of the campus. She acted in two of the dramatic society's plays and auditioned for the lead in one of them. She played on the tennis team for one season and was a candidate for manager of women's varsity softball team in her junior year. One semester she spent several lunches a week with the French club at their special table. But when asked for letters of recommendation, her professors also found themselves in a conflict of feelings. Yes, Sarah's class attendance was excellent. She was always prepared for class and was actively involved in class discussions, but the professors often had problems making sure others had an opportunity to participate because of Sarah's tendency to dominate. Her test scores were always very good, though here too was a problem. On essay questions Sarah wrote more than was asked for by digressing from the question, making the grading of her answers more difficult. Also, she often openly disagreed with her professors' points of view.

In her senior year Sarah put together a résumé of college activities to be included with applications for graduate school or future employement. At a first and superficial reading it was an impressive list of "credits." However, after studying the résumé more thoroughly, one realized that, except for her very good grades, something was missing. Not once did the résum'e show that her peers had selected her to be in a position of leadership. She was never even an assistant editor of the yearbook or newspaper, although she had worked hard and had done some good writing. She was not reelected to the student government after one semester. She was not given a lead part in a play, although she was acknowledged to be a good actress. She was not captain of any team, or even the head manager when she was a candidate for that position. Why was she in the French club for only one semester, when she had a minor in foreign language?

What her résumé did not show was that three of her roommates had changed rooms. For the last two years she lived in a single, and she had no close friends. The reader has to wonder why. What do you think? (A class may pause here and speculate before going on for more information.)

This point was not lost on Sarah either. She had asked herself the same question many times, but insight was not one of her assets. By the time her college years were almost over, she was a frustrated, disillusioned, and lonely girl. At this point, she changed her game plan but not for the better. There was no longer any chance of winning; the only strategy left was not to lose. To anyone maneuvered into listening, she widely projected the blame for her failures on to politics, prejudice, and favoritism. She was heard to say, "Who wants to be in those immature cliquish clubs anyway?" and "I have more important things to do with my time," and "It certainly is a lot less trouble and inconvenience to have a room to myself."

Interviews with some of the people on campus who knew Sarah well provide us with useful insights into the reasons for her failure to be accepted.

Other women in the dorm, especially the three ex-roommates, commented in ways like this: "Life around Sarah was a constant game of one-upmanship. She could always go you one better. Any conversation turned into an argument. She always had to be right. Her opinion was the only one that was correct. Her suggestion was the only one that was acceptable. It was non-negotiable. I don't need being put down all of the time. She always had to be superior, and she was such a snobbish bitch about it."

The faculty producer of the student drama productions made these comments: "Sarah was very difficult to work with. She was constantly disagreeing with the director, and was very uncooperative. She frequently criticized the other actors and even the technical crews. You can't give a lead role to a person like that; it would constantly disrupt the entire show. It's too bad. She had some talent."

The coaches reported similar experiences: "Sarah was one big pain. We were relieved when she didn't come out for the team the next season. She created too much dissension—openly second-guessing the coaches, publicly criticizing the other girls' play and fingering blame if we lost a game. When she was an assistant manager, she spent one whole evening devising a new scoring system that allegedly was to improve the defects in a system that is standard in the league. She was angrily disbelieving when we would not change. She created a lot of enemies on the team."

The editor of the school newspaper, who was an experienced senior, said to the dean after he fired Sarah: "I regretted having to get rid of a hard worker, but in her eyes we weren't doing anything right. You can't have two chief editors on a newspaper, especially when the other one is a green freshman."

She was such a disruptive member of the student government that the dorm had to elect another representative the following semester. She was much too outspoken and aggressive. She had little patience with the democratic process or the majority rule. She had no concept of compromise or acceptance of differing points of view. She singlehandedly came close to causing the French club luncheons to be cancelled for low attendance. Too few students were willing to tolerate her inconsiderate domination of the conversations or her supercritical correcting of other students' minor flaws of pronunciation.

How does a person, especially an intelligent person, become so totally self-focused, to the point of being ignorant of and disinterested in other people's needs? A brief look at Sarah's background may provide some insight.

Sarah was honored with the name of her maternal grandmother, Sarah Winston B. Her grandmother was widely recognized as a brilliant academic and president of a small but prestigious New England girls' school. She was an awesome model to emulate. Sarah's parents were both of a scholarly disposition also. They met when both were working on graduate degrees in English at the same university. Mr. J. was an executive in a large publishing firm, and Mrs. J. was a teacher. Sarah had an older sister, Beatrice, who had successfully followed the lead of her parents with an exceptional academic record. She was already an assistant editor with a book publishing company.

The J. home was neat and orderly with everything in the right place and under control. A first-time guest in their home was made quite comfortably by their gracious, courteous hospitality. People of longer acquaintance would be met with a genuine handshake or a somewhat formal kiss on the cheek, although no relationships ever reached the point of hugging. One intuitively realized that there was a line of intimacy across which one did not step. The J.'s had a number of good friends, but no one listed them among their intimate friends. Within the family there was a strong sense of unity, but it was obligatory and proper rather than emotionally intimate. Strong emotional expression had never been permitted; it would upset the composure and security. Mr. and Mrs. J. were both skilled at intellectualizing emotional issues that might complicate the home atmosphere. Consequently, there was little emotional sharing within the family, even between the parents. Needless to say, the girls received little in the way of love or affection, only approval or disapproval. Sarah, in particular, had no example from which to learn how to understand others' feelings, and certainly no experience with empathy.

The parents assumed such high standards of performance that it was taken for granted. However, praise was hard to come by; a perfunctory acknowledgment was the norm. It was difficult for Sarah ever to know whether her efforts to please were successful. It is ironic that a girl whose natural aptitudes included an ample measure of intelligence and competence should grow up in constant struggle with a sense of inferiority. Superiority is relative to the standards set for comparison.

While some background knowledge about the child helps us to better understand the personality and behavior of the young adult, we are left with one last perplexing question about Sarah's behavior. You may have asked it a number of times about the behavior of maladjusted people you have known. it usually takes one of these forms: "Why does he keep doing the same stupid things over and over again? He must be able to see that he's making things worse in the long run." or "Why doesn't she think in this logical and reasonable way instead of that crazy, irrational way? It doesn't make any sense." In short, why are nonintegrative, "bad" adjustments repeated? Shaffer and Shoben call it the "adjustment paradox." Paradox means self-contradiction; that is, an adjustment that is not an adjustment.

Confused? Here's how it applies to a case like Sarah's. First, all behavior, even "stupid" behavior, is motivated. What was Sarah's primary motivation? It certainly seemed that dominant among her needs was her social motivation.

She appeared to be trying desperately to show people how terrific she was so that she would receive recognition, approval, and acceptance. Her method for achieving this included a variety of behaviors that loudly announced, "I'm the best, I'm the greatest, I can do anything better than anyone." She continued to use this style of adjustive behavior for years. How did her peers and others react to this behavior? Quite predictably: "Oh, no, you're not. And, furthermore, we don't like you or your style, and we don't want you in our group." Then why did she keep doing those things? This kind of behavior contradicts one of the basic tenets of psychology—Thorndike's law of effect. This states, roughly, that "successful" responses tend to be repeated (and are thus said to be reinforced) and "unsuccessful" responses tend to be discarded. The law of effect is the basis for the learning principle of operant conditioning, also called instrumental conditioning.

Thus, the repetition of punished behavior probably doesn't make any sense to us. It seems to say that the principle of operant conditioning is wrong. How do we resolve the paradox?

In Sarah's case we must go back and reexamine our initial assumptions. When Sarah seemed to be trying so hard to impress people with her superiority, was it really other people that she most needed to convince? If not, who?

What can we infer from our answer about the true nature of Sarah's self-concept? This hypothesis is a reasonable one to consider whenever we are trying to understand someone who seems to be "overdoing it," trying too hard to convince other of toughness, or masculinity, or honesty, or loyalty, for example. Remember the famous line from Shakespeare's *Hamlet*, "The lady doth protest too much, methinks."

QUESTIONS FOR DISCUSSION

1. How do you *feel* when someone's behavior makes you feel inferior? How do you *react?*
2. Does your "punishment" of the individual help the situation, or solve the problem?
3. Can you think of the male counterpart of the Sarah personality and how he would behave in the get-acquainted period of freshman year? How would his fellow students react to him?
4. Would you judge Sarah's social motivation to be high or low? (Social needs are needs for approval, acceptance, belonging, love, etc.)
5. What criteria do you use when voting for a president, captain, or any other leader of an organization you belong to? Would you vote to make Sarah your captain or president? Why or why not?
6. Did Sarah really feel as superior to everyone as she acted? What was the true nature of her self-concept?
7. What are the most important ingredients of a positive self-concept? Did Sarah have any of these?

Chapter
4

The Escape and
Avoid Choice

BILL O.: I'M VERY HAPPY HERE IN MY ROOM

Introduction

In Chapter 3 we discussed the two basic choices of response to personal threat, and considered how the fight choice can be carried to a degree which results in maladjustment.

Now we turn to the opposite option, whereby a person finds ways to escape from personal danger and devises mechanisms for avoiding any future encounters with the threat.

It is important to state at the outset that I am not saying that one or the other of these choices is better or preferable. In fact, either can be the wiser course of action depending on the circumstances. While our culture generally approves and encourages us to stand up and defend ourselves with courage and "guts," and not be a "wimp" or a "sissy," it sometimes is a much wiser tactic to hold back and be submissive if the confronter is more powerful or dangerous. For example, if a police officer is about to give you a warning for speeding, or an angry parent wants to discuss your duties and priviliges, or a superior officer in the military takes exception to your appearance in a humiliating manner. To repeat, the healthy personality is notable for its flexibility and the absence of rigid, unchanging habits.

I believe it is particularly important to understand the good and bad aspects of the flight option, because it seems to have become, over the last few decades, increasingly the preferred choice for adolescents, in this critical learning period during which they establish the mechanisms for coping with life in adulthood. Teenagers have discovered a great variety of ways to postpone dealing with problems or to pretend they do not exist. For example:

alcohol, marijuana, cocaine, and other brain-affecting drugs, mind-numbing loud noise, "cruising" and partying, fantasy, or even just lots of sleeping. This trend is of serious concern to psychologists because ignored decisions and problems seldom just go away, as one would like to hope. They stay and accumulate, making life ever more complicated and overwhelming in the long run. Furthermore, the young person may be postponing, possibly until too late, the learning of good problem-solving skills, which will be necessary in order to become an independent, productive adult.

To understand this flight choice more thoroughly, it is helpful to reexamine the fight/flight option from a different perspective—a somewhat more technical one. Most life problems that a person perceives as personally threatening result from conflict. A conflict is a situation in which you want two or more things at the same time, but are forced to choose only one. Refer to your textbooks on introductory or adjustment psychology for a more detailed discussion of the dynamics of the different kinds of conflict. The most difficult and stressful kind of conflict problem to solve is called an approach–avoidance conflict. This is a situation where a single goal is attractive or needed, but at the same time causes negative, unpleasant feelings such as fear or anxiety. Think of a $1,000 bill lying in a nest of poisonous snakes. The most popular paradigm that psychologists use to illustrate an approach–avoidance conflict is shown in Figure 4.1.

I have selected, as a specific example, a common difficult conflict, which can be used to illustrate the fight/flight choice. We start with the assumption that almost everyone has strong needs for the approval, acceptance, and being liked and loved that other people provide. These motivate us to seek the company of other people and join in their activities. For some people, especially the overly defensive person who was described in Chapter 3, this impulse toward social interaction will be inhibited by fear of rejection, criticism, humiliation, or embarassment. A conflict exists when these opposing impules are at equal strength, and the person only can vacillate in indecision.

The only way to resolve a conflict is to make the opposing impulses unequal by changing one's perception of the situation in some way. In the fight choice, the person strengthens the adient or approach impulse by aggressive-

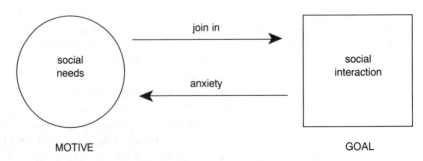

Figure 4.1. The approach–avoidance conflict.

ly asserting his acceptability and superiority. At the same time, he weakens the ability of others to hurt him by attacking them first, as Sarah did. A person disposed to making flight choices would handle the situation differently. He or she would weaken the adient impluse by denying its importance. This denial would leave the impulse to escape and avoid social situations the stronger one and it would tend to prevail. So the person is more comfortable simply not giving others the opportunity to cause pain. "They can't reject me if I stay away from them." "I can't flunk the test if I find a way not to take it." "The dog can't bite me if I don't try to pet it."

To illustrate how an uncompromising tendency to depend on escape and avoidance mechanisms to cope with social threat can result in maladjustment, consider the following case.

The Saga of Suzie and Bill

It is the first psychology class of the first semester of the college year. An attractive freshman named Suzie is chatting amiably with some of her new friends from the dorm, waiting for class to start. She is outgoing and friendly and is enjoying the independence and challenges and the new social life at the beginning of college. As the professor calls the class to order, she begins to "check out" the other kids in the class. She notices across the room near the front of the class a "cute" guy concentrating on copying down some preliminary information that the teacher is writing on the chalkboard. Almost immediately, she decides that she is going to give this fortunate "fish" the opportunity and privilege of getting to know her. When the professor checks the attendance by calling out names from the class roster, Suzie takes care to note that the name of the target is William O. At the end of class, Bill has disappeared by the time she can make her way to that side of the room to try to start a conversation. But, by the next class, she has planned her strategy for hooking this trout. By timing it carefully, she manages to sit in the seat right beside him, where attention getting will be made easier. With her stylishly short miniskirt, knees crossed in his direction, foot twitching, a little bit of extra cologne, she set the lure. But Bill didn't seem to notice. Guess the trout aren't feeding today. At the end of the class she "accidentally" knocked her books on the floor, so that Bill had to pick them up before he could get out of his seat, and this he did. "Thank you," she said, sweetly. "You're welcome," he mumbled quietly, not looking directly into her face. Then he walked out of the classroom. "Well, what's with this guy anyway?" she thought. She decided to give him one more chance. The next day she sat in the same seat and made additional efforts to get his attention, but he still would not look at her for more than a second or two. At the end of the class she asked him a direct question. "Did you hear what the teacher said about the homework?" "Have chapter 1 read by Friday." Bill replied awkwardly, as if embarrassed. And he walked out of the room again. "That's it," decided Suzie, "there are other fish in the pond. What is this guy's problem anyway? I don't need all this rejection."

What is Bill's problem? (A class may stop here and speculate before reading on for more information.)

Bill O. was the only child of Irish-American parents. The family had always lived in a quiet neighborhood where there were few other children, and none near his age. He become accustomed to being alone and finding solitary kinds of activities, because there were no siblings or other neighborhood children to play with. He was a bright boy and found much pleasure in various collections—bugs, baseball cards, stamps, and coins. He acquired reading skills early, and by the time he was 10 he had become an avid reader of adventure books. His active imagination enabled him to fill the gaps in his real-life experience with fantasy. Bill's grade school teachers described him as a "nice boy," a "good boy," and absolutely no trouble to have in class—always polite and cooperative, perhaps a little too quiet and unassertive, not apt to stick up for himself with more aggressive boys even when they called him "wimpy" names. They allowed that he was a bit too much of a "mama's boy," even though he had good reason to be and had trouble doing anything about it. By the time he was in late junior high and high school, the teachers described his personality in similar ways but in stronger terms. They used language like "in a shell," withdrawn, seclusive, no social skills with peers, self-conscious, and not at ease. In fact, he had been referred for sessions with one of the school counselors.

Mrs. O. ran the home in a conscientious, well-intended but overly serious manner. Her conscientiousness was carried to the extreme and she was an overdominant and overprotective mother. Some described her as having a "quick flaring Irish temper"–which meant that to defy her was to risk the wrath of demons. She had strong and firm opinions, which tended to be highly moralistic. "Bad" and "sinful" were not uncommon words in her vocabulary. Bill's difficulty in learning social skills was exacerbated by his mother's insistent overinvolvement in his life. She made him wear a raincoat and rubbers to school if there was even a suggestion of bad weather. She made him come home for lunch instead of letting him eat in the school's perfectly satisfactory cafeteria with the other kids. She even came to pick him up and return him to school if it rained. Although schools generally want parents to show interest in their children's progress, Mrs. O.'s frequent contact with the office and the teachers was excessive to the pont of being a "pest." Bill found it a much easier course of action to simply give in and humor her, in order to avoid the hassle and keep the peace. His mother's sarcasm and highly moralistic personal criticism were too high a price to pay for resisting.

Mr. O. was a hardworking salesman who was well liked and respected by his associates. He was generally thought by those who knew him to be a "nice guy." His work required him to be away from home much of the week. This was unfortunate from Bill's perspective, because his dad was his hero and pal whom he loved and admired. For Bill he was the only source of hugs and genuine personal attention. It was a relief when his father was home to share in coping with his mother's temperament. However, Mr.O. was no match for his wife's strong, agressive personality either. He also maintained a passive

THE SAGA OF SUZIE AND BILL   25

role in the home "to keep the peace." And because Mr. O. was from a strong religious background, he seldom interfered with his wife's excessive moralizing, although he too was uncomfortable with it. Mr. and Mrs. O. did little socializing as a couple, except for church-centered activites.

The long-range possibilities for a successful social adjustment for Bill were worsened by events and experiences that happened when he was in the eighth and ninth grades. Several things combined to reinforce his preference for protective isolation and seclusiveness. First, when Bill was 13, his father abruptly and without warning left the home. Mr. O., to his own surprise, had fallen in love with a "warm and gentle" woman who made him consciously aware of his long-term deprivation of a comfortable intimacy. So he simply moved out and went to live with the other woman.

Following this upheaval , the atmosphere in Bill's home went from uncomfortable to intolerable. Many boys survive, psychologically, the loss of a father, but for Bill it was different—his only trustworthy source of love had betrayed him. Although his father insisted that he still loved Bill, it was difficult to have any time together. In the little time when his father was not traveling, the new woman also had expectations on his time. And following their infrequent days together, Bill dreaded returning hom to his mother's angry raving about his father's infidelity and that "whore he lives with," and the interminable awkward questions. In addition were the severe financial strains. Mr. O. was limited in the amount of support money he could send. Mrs. O., with few salable skills, had to go to work for a housecleaning business. Many single mothers have had to support the home in such ways, but Mrs. O. never let Bill forget her "sacrifice" and travail of "working my fingers to the bone." Any attempt by Bill to venture into social activities, especially those that might cost money, was met with a heavy load of guilt, and accusations of his "ingratitude" and "wastefulness."

In the ninth grade, adolescent urgings induced Bill to become smitten with a girl in his homeroom. When she surprisingly showed return interest, he took the risk of spending as much time as he could with her during the school day, talking and sharing ideas and feelings. After a few weeks, during which Bill considered her his "girl friend," the girl became bored with his shyness, immaturity, and unwillingness to go out at night; she dropped him for a more "mature" boy who was a year older. Bill suffered another devastating betrayal of trust.

In the same year he acquired a pal who had similar interests, and for that year they were "best friends." In fact, each was the only real friend the other one had. Each was the confidant for the other's most personal concerns. In the week before school was over for that year Bill's friend, Ray, was killed instantly in an automobile accident caused by a speeding drunk driver. Bill took no more risks of intimacy during his high school years. He had a job to help with expenses, and he studied for a scholarship to college. He was lonely and he had many fantasies, but he wasn't hurt again. He was also, as a senior, years behind his peers in social skills and sophistication.

QUESTIONS FOR DISCUSSION

1. When Suzie tried to "toss the ball" to Bill, did he see it coming?
2. Can you label the approach–avoidance conflict that Bill is in when Suzie presents her "opportunity"? Concentrate on the negative or inhibition impluse.
3. What do you think is the future prognosis for Bill's social adjustment?
4. DWhat would be required to help him, or do you think it is too late? (Hint: What would you suggest or do to help a friend who had a phobia of dogs?)
5. What kind of factors or experiences do you think are involved in predisposing a person to prefer escape adjustments rather than more (socially) aggressive ones?
6. What is the role of repression in helping "flight" mechanisms to be successful in reducing anxiety?

Chapter
5
Phobia
A Symbolic Escape

MARIA D.: THE FANGS OF GUILT

Introduction

Do you have any phobias? What are you afraid of: spiders, snakes, the dark, being up high, ambulance sirens? Do you feel a little queasiness in the stomach, a tightness in your chest, do you have sweaty hands, pounding heart, difficulty breathing, even a little dizziness? The psychology of fear causes any or all of these sensations. Do you feel a little self-conscious and foolish, too embarrassed to tell anyone about it if you can help it? Do you have certain planned habits or rituals for avoiding certain things? Then maybe you do have a phobia. You need not be self-conscious, for a great number of people do. It may be "normal." The National Institute of Mental Health (NIMH) estimates that perhaps 20 million people suffer from phobias. Some experts even believe that almost everyone has at least minor phobias. But maybe you don't. Perhaps it is just a strong fear that is quite reasonable, depending on how you acquired it. We all have had experiences with fire, or vicious dogs, or being under water, or ambulance sirens, or automobile accidents—so terrifying we want to avoid those things because they make us recall the awful original experience. But a strong fear is not necessarily a phobia. Phobia is another of those words that gets bandied about in the vernacular much too freely.

Phobia is a clinical, technical term. It means unreasonable or irrational fear. Phobias are irrational for two reasons: (1) The fear reaction is excessive relative to the real threat or danger in the situation. (2) The person also does not know why he or she is afraid and cannot explain it. Phobics often feel quite embarrassed and foolish, yet cannot control the feeling. Most times we can remember quite well when and how we acquired our normal fears.

Like ordinary fears, phobias happen in all degrees of severity, from mild uneasiness to uncontrollable panic. But the common ingredient is irrationality. The feelings are very real indeed but the phobic stimulus makes no sense. In fact, sometimes there is no specific stimulus at all. The awful fear is spontaneous and unfocused. "I don't know why, I just suddenly feel afraid and panicky, and I can't help it." At the extreme, phobias are such an intense uncontrollable state of panic, and occur so frequently, that the person's life is reduced to almost total ineffectiveness. Each day is dominated by the desperate need to avoid whatever is causing the anxiety. The compulsive avoidance rituals generalize to more and more places, and the safe world becomes smaller and smaller. Needless to say, this behavior can also seriously affect the lives of any other people who live with the phobic person.

To understand what it is like to be phobic, try this exercise. Imagine that you are locked in a small room or closet. There is no light. Think of something that causes you revulsion—perhaps spiders and snakes. Imagine that there are a hundred of these locked in the dark room with you. Allright, that's enough, come back to reality. At least *you* can do it at will. Now perhaps you can appreciate how somes lives become so disrupted and dominated by a phobia.

Phobia is a Greek word meaning, of course, "fear of." It is traditional simply to take the Greek word for the feared thing and attach phobia to the end of it. Because a person can develop a phobia about anything, given the right circumstances, there can be no definitive list of them. However, it is worth mentioning a few that are common or interesting.

Claustrophobia is fear of enclosed places, for example, elevators.

Agoraphobia is the fear of open places. Agoraphobia also can have a more complicated, broader meaning, for in Greek it means fear of the marketplace, which implies a situation that is busy and crowded with people.

Acrophobia is fear of heights.

Triskaidekaphobia is fear of the number 13.

Hydrophobia is fear of water.

Zoophobia is the fear of animals.

Phobia has always been a somewhat mysterious disorder and a conundrum for clinical psychology and psychiatry. Many of the old questions remain: Why do frightening experiences for children turn into adult phobias for some people but not for others? Why are they more common in women (at least twice as frequent)? Are the causes mainly psychological, or do the brains of phobics have a different biochemistry? What is the best kind of therapy to cure a phobia? Despite its mysteries, clinicians do seem to be making some progress. As with the other "abnormalities" that have historically been most troublesome for psychiatry (e.g., schizophrenia, manic-depression, alcoholism), there is now strong research evidence that phobic thinking and behavior may be partly caused by abnormal biochemistry in the brain. Furthermore, there may be a hereditary predisposition for this.

But we are studying psychology, and out task is simply to allow for the biological variables, while continuing to pursue a better understanding of the psychological dynamics of a problem. This attempt to clarify our understanding is reflected in a recent change in the way the American Psychiatric Association puts phobias into different categories. In the *DSM IIIR*, there are three categories: simple phobia, agoraphobia, and social phobia. I still do not find this a particularly useful system because the three categories are not mutally exclusive. In fact, there is a great deal of overlapping between them.

It is useful, however, to discuss phobia as a single phenomenon, even if that is an oversimplification, because it provides us with some insights into how the mind works—especially when it is not working in a very healthy fashion.

COMMON FEATURES OF PHOBIAS

Let's take a brief look at what clinical case histories over the years have to tell us about common factors in the experiences of phobic individuals. First, phobias most often can be traced back to a very frightening experience (or experiences) that happened in childhood. The adult usually cannot remember this experience, or at least not some important details of the experience. The reason he or she cannot remember the event is that it has been repressed. This is the essential psychological ingredient of a phobia. Recall is repressed because something about the experience is threatening to self-esteem. For example, the child may have been doing something "bad," or "naughty," or forbidden. This may be why it often appears as if the person's "child" is in control during the irrational fearful reaction. It is not uncommon for others to remember that the phobic person was an insecure "'fraidy cat" as a child. In the simpler forms the stimuli for a phobic reaction has a direct connection with the original frightening but forgotten experience. For example, a boy was chased and terrified by a snarling dog when he was trespassing in a yard where he had been forbidden to go and threatened with punishment if he did. Naturally, he didn't tell anyone about the experience and he eventually repressed the memory of the experience to avoid "bad boy" anxiety feelings. In later years he learns he is more comfortable if he stays away from dogs, although he does not understand why. Similar things can happen with close or high places, running water, fire, etc.

As unusual as it may seem, because phobias are so unpleasant, they can actually be considered adjustment mechanisms in that they provide prople with some measure of control, by avoidance, over anxieties they do not consciously understand. Thus, they are a kind of symbolic escape. The boy's staying away from dogs avoids feelings of guilt.

There is another variety of phobias that is apt to be even more adjustive. They are more complicated and even more symbolic. In fact, I call them "symbolic" phobias, in contrast to "simple" phobias. The most difficult kinds of threat to cope with are those that are abstract—only ideas or concepts, not real things. There are fairly clear choices of what you can do about bears or mean dogs or bullies or lightning storms. But what do you do about the "boogie man" who was everywhere in the dark, or feelings of guilt, or helplessness, or failure, or fear of death? You can't run away from these personal anxieties; they follow right along with you. They are faceless and formless and, for some people, lurk everywhere. What the mind tries to do is to find a concrete form to attach them to, so that there is something to shoot at, or hit, or run away from. This is what the mind is doing is some of our strange dreams and nightmares. In symbolic phobias the mind discovers something concrete that stands for and takes the place of the abstract anxiety, and attaches the feelings to it. The person develops habits and rituals for avoiding the feared thing, and in this way manages to keep the anxiety under control. All of this behavior goes on unconsciously. The person doesn't understand the reason for avoiding this thing, only that he or she feels better doing it.

I once knew a women who was brought reluctantly for psychotherapy by her husband. He had reached a point of total frustration and despair over the amount of home disruption and family tension caused by two pattersn of compulsive phobic behavior. The first one was about flies. The home was an arsenal of fly traps, insect sprays, and fly swatters. The appearance of any form of fly, but particularly common houseflies, triggered instant mobilization of the weapons, and distraction from any other ongoing task—it was as if the home were being invaded by the devil. The second was a system of prophylactic rituals and nightly examinations to detect and prevent the slightest indication of the presence of pin worms or other intestinal parasites, which are a common and medically unimportant occurence in children.

In the course of therapy, two long "forgotten" experiences of her childhood were recalled. Evidently she had been a somewhat insecure but spoiled and willful little girl. On one occassion, when she was being "mischievous," an older relative, who was of a highly fundamentalist religious persuasion, pointed a bony finger at her and declared emphatically, "You are going to rot in hell if you don't stop being a bad girl!" The second event occurred while she was walking in a field and happened upon the body of a dead animal. She found the sight of a nest of maggots consuming the carcass totally repulsive. Years later, in late adolescence, when her maturing brain began to be able to contemplate the abstracts of soul, infinity, death, and eternity, she developed a recurring anxiety about dying. It was anchored in the long-repressed warning threat from her religious relative. The magnificent computer that is the brain searched its memory banks for something concrete to represent this vague fear. Unfortunately it came upon the image of the worms consuming the dead body. The phobia generalized to flies later, when she learned that maggots are the larvae that develop from fly eggs. Thus, an all-out attack on flies and their larvae enabled this woman to feel some degree of direct control over the vague fear of death.

The details of another case illustrate the clever way the mind can use symbols to help it cope with complicated forms of threat.

The Case of Maria D.

I came to know Maria as a member of a therapy group. She was a young woman in her thirties of Italian heritage. She was married for less than two years
and had a young son about one year old. She was slightly overweight, but
always neatly dressed and carefully made up. She tended to be a little shy,
self-conscious, and quiet. Her manner was pleasant, courteous, and proper,
but a little intense and excitable. She was always punctual—in fact, usually
early—for the meetings, and always sat in the same chair.

For the first several sessions of the weekly meetings, the group did not
know much about Maria. In her unassertive way she tended to defer to others
who had a greater need to talk about themselves. We knew that she had
married fairly late, relative to the traditional Italian family pattern. We knew
also that she had entered therapy mostly at her husband's insistence, although
she herself was initially reluctant. His concerns apparently were that marriage
and parenting were very stressful for her, and she was "driving him crazy."
She was an overanxious mother, always worried that something would happen
to the child (like getting sick form poisoned food), and was much too overprotective. She had to be "very careful" about the baby's food. It had to be
smelled and tasted several times before she would feed it to him—in case it
was tainted. Much "good" food was thrown out and wasted. She hovered over
the baby like a "mother hen," fearful that he would bump or hurt himself, or
put something "dirty" in his mouth. Her husband, Tony, complained that, for
Maria, "cleaning" came close to sterilizing. It was unreasonable to be expected to live in an "operating room" where he was afraid to touch anything.
On the occasion when Tony suggested getting a puppy as a pet for the boy, he
was taken aback by the intensity of Maria's arguments against the idea. For
some reason she felt that dogs were "dirty and dangerous." There were also
indications, from her remarks, that there was less than ideal compatibility between them in their sexual relations. Having a headache was only one of many
excuses she used. She confessed that it was "difficult for her to relax." She
made this statement ruefully. Maria wanted very much to be a "good wife."
She regarded it as her most important life role and duty. It was the fact that
she felt her tensions were causing her to fall short of this goal that she agreed
to go for help—"if it will make Tony happy." "He tries to be patient, but is a
lusty and emotional man." "He is good about taking showers at night when I
ask him."

These spotty details, revealed over a period of time, were enough to satisfy the group that Maria had reason to be in the therapy group, but there was
no further searching for insights into any deeper or more serious neuroses. So
the group was therefore surprised by the events that took place about the
tenth week of the therapy sessions. It was obvious that something was wrong
when Maria was not in her accustomed seat at the start of the meeting. The
group occupied itself for more than a few minutes speculating as to whether
Maria may have dropped out.

Thus, the group was startled when, some 15 or 20 minutes into the meeting, Maria burst through the door, out of breath, perspiring, her hair and

clothing disheveled, and her face colorless and terrified. There was instant mutual understanding in the group htat Maria would do most of the talking this afternoon. Responding to this patient acceptance and her own need, she did indeed talk, and talk, and talk. No she had not witnessed a horrible automobile accident, nor had her baby been rushed to the hospital, nor had she been molested by a street mugger. She had merely confronted a dog on the sidewalk as she walked to the clinic. Unable to proceed without coming closer to the beast, she retreated in panic and, running as much of the time as she could, had detoured several blocks out of her way in order to avoid the animal. To make matters worst, this was the second time in two days that she had been confronted by a dog. The previous evening she had gone to visit friends, not knowing they had a new pet dog. Just as she closed the front door behind her the dog came into the hallway to investigate. Maria was trapped. She screamed in terror and nearly climbed the wall in panic to the complete consernation and embarrassment of her hosts. The dog had to be locked in the garage before she would agree to stay. Until this time the therapy group was unaware of her phobia.

Maria's talking, during that meeting, was highly emotional and subjective. It was rambling and disconnected. There was seldom a consistent train of thought for any length of time that could be followed logically. Because the meeting ended shortly after she ran out of talk, it was some time later before I was able to sort out the important details. As I saw it, the psychologically significant details of her life story were these: Maria's immigrant parents were simple, uneducated, honest, and hardworking. They had a very conservative religious morality. As a result, Maria, their only daughter, was brought up sheltered, overprotected, and naive. The most significant event occurred when she was 11. On the morning after Maria's menarche arrived, Mrs. D. sat her down for the *Talk*. Instead of being understanding or consoling, she dealt very matter-of-factly with Maria's inital shock and fear that she was "bleeding to death," and proceeded with the short-form sex education lesson. The Mrs. D. version consisted of the following five rules:

1. This is the beginning of your becoming a woman. You may begin to feel a different interest in boys, and even have sexual thoughts.
2. It is naughty, bad, even sinful to have any physical contact with men before you are married. "Good" girls do not do such things; they do not even think about such things.
3. All men are "beasts." They have only one thing on their minds. Watch out for them. Do not trust them.
4. Don't forget that your father is also a man. So from now on don't be alone with him!
5. After you are married, sex is OK. In fact, it is your duty to satisfy your husband's wishes.

This set of "rules," offered often by well-meaning but ignornat parents to "protect" their teenage daughters, has caused many psychological problems by creating troublesome sexual conflicts and minor neuroses in countless young women through the generations. It is difficult or impossible for a young woman suddenly to change her attitude to sex is OK or even "beautiful" on her wedding day, when she had been taught to believe all through her adolescent years that sex was bad or sinful. But, poor Maria. This naive 11-year-old had been burdened not only with a difficult sexual conflict as her sexuality matured, but also with a second cruel conflict—ambivalent feelings toward her father, whom she had always loved.

This case is an interesting example of how the mind can atempt to revolve difficult and poorly understood conflicts by symbolic displacement. It seems that a key element in both of Maria's conflicts was the concept of men as "beasts." So her mind selected the dog as a representative beast on which symbolically to focus her anxieties. I do not know how this happened. She may well have seen dogs copulating when she was a girl, or observed her mother reacting with anger or disgust at such an event. At any rate, while Maria could not run away from her ambivalent feelings, she could achieve some control over anxiety by avoiding dogs.

To return to our general discussion of phobias, there is one last question to consider. I will mention it only briefly, even though it is a broad question. If any of you go on into training in clinical psychology, you will encounter controversy or uncertainty regarding the best treatment for phobias. Currently, there are three. In historical sequence, they are: insight psychotherapy, behavior therapy, and chemotherapy or medication. All three have strong advocates. Let me suggest this thought as a resolution to the question. Any one, or a combination, may be the best treatment, depending on the case. Clearly there are at least three predisposing factors to one's becoming phobic: a greater than normal tendency to use repression as an adjustment mechanism, poor adjustment learning in general (nonintegrative adjustment habits), and abnormal brain chemistry. Therefore, a careful determination of the cause of a given problem is needed, in order to prescribe the optimal therapy or combination of therapies. I emphasize the word careful, because there are cases when a treatment that only deals with symptoms can be psychologically dangerous.

QUESTIONS FOR DISCUSSION

1. Can you imagine an example of phobia in which something even as simple as a particular name evokes anxiety and avoidance?
2. Can you diagram the approach–avoidance conflicts that are at the core of Maria's neurosis, as you did in Chapter 4?
3. How would you have handled the situation if you were Maria's husband? What are his options?
4. What do you think is the long-term prognosis for Maria's marriage? Will the couple be able to save it?

Chapter
6
Hysteria
Adjustment Through Disability

NANCY L.: YOU HAVE TO CONSIDER MY CONDITION

Introduction: A Third Variety of Escape Mechanism

Do you remember when you were a kid and you said to your mother, "Mommy, I don't feel good today"? And your mother very likely said, "OK honey, you'd better not go to shcool today. You just stay in bed." How nice it was to have an easy day of being pampered and "taken care of." Maybe this special consideration was even useful later on, when there was an assignment not ready or a test not prepared for, or some other situation at school that you did not want to deal with. It is an easy lesson to lear—that society excuses us from responsibilities when we are sick. Many people bring this knowledge into adulthood with them. In a modern industrial society, most companies provide a certain number of paid sick day, and their employees usually find a way to use them. Some of these "days out" are well justified—even it they are only occasional reviving "mental health days." If we add the occurrences of the famous "headache" or upset stomach or menstrual discomfort, we have enough medical excuses for getting out of anxiety-laden social situations to make the phenomenon common enough to be called normal. This is not pathology, although, it may often be irresponsibility, or "chickening out."

However, as we move up the continuum of quality of adjustment into the neurotic range, we find some psychological phenomena that definitely are not normal. In fact, they represent some of the most bizarre and interesting cases in all of clinical psychology. They actually predate by thousands of years any formal science or profession of psychology. They have presented a baffling kind of problem for physicians for as long as there has been a written history of medicine. These cases presented themselves to physicians for treatment, but doctors could find nothing medical or physiological to treat. They represented all kinds of ailments or disabilities, and some were truly disabling. They may have taken the form of blindness when there was nothing wrong with the eyes, or deafness when there was nothing wrong with the hearing mechanism. There may have been loss of feeling on localized parts of the body, or painful cramping or muscle spasms, or full paralysis of an arm or leg— but thee was nothing wrong with the neurology of these parts. Sometimes the condition was chronic and sometimes it occurred in only certain situations— when the pianist had to play the piano, when the typist had to type, or when the singer had to sing, although each could perform other tasks with the afflicted part.

Over a long period of time, as we gradually learned how the brain works, we began to understand what was going on. In some individuals the mind simply decides to reclaim the special consideration given to the sick child. When confronted with a difficult conflict or social expectation, they simply get sick or disabled. It may be spontaneous, like a paralysis, or a continuation of a disabling condition, such as laryngitis, which had really existed earlier as part of a cold. It is their visable "note from the doctor" stating, "I'm obviously too sick to play in the game today"—and begging to be excused. "You really can't expect me to perform in my condition."

You should not get the idea that these people are malingering or "faking it." They could not tolerate the guilt or social criticism if this were the case. They truly believe in their disabilities. They truly cannot feel, or see, or hear, or use that arm. Their condition is similar to a highly suggestible hypnotic state. The mind uses its incredible capacity to inhibit reponse or awareness through repression. It is a terrifically effective adjustment. The person gets out of a difficult conflict situation and is provided with a guilt-free rationalization. But that is not all.

Additional reinforcement for this adjustment mechanism comes from what we call *secondary gains.* These are additional benefits—frosting the cake, so to speak. Being sick also usually results in attention and sympathy and being "taken care of." The patient is also able to manipulate and control other people; sometimes it even includes compensation—being paid while not working.

The name we use to describe these strange afflictions is *hysteria,* or hysterical ailments. I've never been able to discover where the name came from. It is another of those traditional medical labels, the origin of which is lost in time which really ought to be replaced, but we haven't come up with a better one. Hysteria—from the Greek word meaning womb—is a misleading label for obvious reasons. The common use of the word calls to mind the stereotyped, excessively emotional screaming woman or raging man. In clinical usage a hysterical person is almost the opposite, a frequently emotionally shallow person with little outward concern regarding his or her disabled condition.

A more modern term, which is sometimes used synonymously, is "dissociative disorders," or just "dissociation." This is a better label, because the person sometimes appears to have dissociated himself from a part of his body or consciousness. Shaffer and Shoben reported an interesting example of this. It describes the case of a young woman standing beside the bed of her dying father, and feeling deep sadness. When the attending physician, a handsome young doctor, came in to check on the patient, the outside of their thighs accidentally brushed together. The young woman was erotically excited by this encounter, but immediately felt guilty about the feelings under the circumstances. Shortly thereafter, she developed an anesthesia or total loss of feeling on the outside of her thigh. Thus, she dissociated herself from the offending part of her body and effectively prevented a recurrence of the inappropriate and untimely reaction. Dissociation is also a useful and appropriate way to describe the psychological dynamics of the more extreme forms of hysteria. These are the dramatic, famous cases of amensia (or fugue) and multiple personality. In both of these situations, there is an extraordinary, massive use of repression to prevent awareness or recall of huge sections of memory and personal history, including one's identity—or else separate patterns of personality, which take over the person's functioning for periods of time.

You should certainly not think of hysteria as a convenient way to get out of some of life's difficult situations. Not everyone can pull off this degree of self-deception. Hysterics tend to be poorly integrated personalities, often immature, naive, and suggestible. And they are obviously able to use repression to a degree that is psychologically very unhealthy. Also, the cost is great. In return for temporarily solving a problem, the person pays the price of loss of a great deal of normal life functioning and personal freedom.

I acknowledge, however, that is is entirely nromal for the child in all of us periodically to try to convince ourselves that "I'm too sick" to get up this morning, or to take that test, or to keep that dentist appointment, or to go to work, or to do that studying tonight. Sometimes the child succeeds, and we usually regret it later; at other times the parent regains control and keeps us from having to pay the consequences. When I had been teaching for about five or six years, an event happened that is less likely to occur today. I was about to give a class a test one morning, when one of the girls came up to my desk to announce that I would have to excuse her from taking the test that day because she had just gotten her period. Well, I was not about to get caught playing God on that one and risk being sexist or insensitive. I simply said "OK, you decide. But remember the makeup test will be Monday morning and it will be all essays," much harder than the multiple-choice test I was about to give. It took her very little time to decide that her condition wasn't so disabling after all. You may have noticed how different people handle such discomforts as colds, hangovers, and injuries. Some perceive them as problems to work through; others use them as excuses to be absent.

In psychology textbooks, we tend to discuss clincial case examples as if they were always simple and clear. In actual practice, it is often difficult and tricky, even for physicians and psychologists, to distinguish hysterical ailments from real ailments, and from real psychosomatic symptoms of stress, such as migraine headaches, gastrointestinal disorders, and so forth. This is particularly true in the early phase of assessment. Hysteria is such a contradiction to "common sense" that we are not predisposed to think of diagnosis.

A good example of this point—and one of the most interesting cases of hysteria that I have ever encountered—follows.

The Case of Nancy L.

Nancy L. was never an ordinary student. She did not emerge from the indistinguishable pack gradually, as usually is the case. Nancy stood out from the first time she walked into my class, with the aid of her white cane to compensate for her visual impairment. She also stood out from the average student because she chose to sit in the front, and listened with rapt attention to every "pearl of wisdom" that emerged from the professor's lips. She also was an attractive young woman, with a sparkling and friendly personality. In addition, I spent extra hours of contact in order to administer oral examinations, and to help her obtain a copy of the textbook on audiotape. During our second course in the spring semester it became necessary to schedule several counseling sessions for adjustment problems indirectly related to her blindness. Another blind student shared some of these sessions. The plot thickened during parents' weekend, when I met Nancy's mother for the first time, and discovered that I had known her 20 years earlier in the course of community service. All in all, by the end of her freshman year, Nancy had become one of the "special people." There was a similar relationship between Nancy and Mrs. C., the caring and able woman who was Nancy's program director.

One of Nancy's personal problems that she shared with both of us was the loneliness of being separated from her boyfriend back home, who was also blind. It was difficult for her to be totally dependent on other people to arrange for them to be together. But actually, all things considered, Nancy's college experience was going successfully. Her academic work was satisfactory, and she even managed to be involved in two student choral groups. She had a beautiful singing voice.

In the fall semester of her second year, I had only occasional and friendly contact with Nancy; she was no longer a student of mine. I kept apprised of her progress via my faculty colleague, Mrs. C. It was in the course of one of these conversations, early in the spring semester, that I was distressed to learn that Nancy revealed to a few people that she was pregnant. There was considerable pessimism expressed between Mrs. C. and me, as we wondered how Nancy would manage this big problem. How would she take care of this child, let alone suport them both? She and her boyfriend were both a long way from completing their educations. Her mother, a widow, was already under financial strain. And Nancy was evidently far enough along in the pregnancy that abortion was not an option. We were also aware that the relationship with the boyfriend had been weakening for some time, rather than growing stronger. We continued to worry through that semester, as we watched her figure gradually assume more fullness of pregnancy.

The whole situation came to a dramatic climax during the week following spring break. On Wednesday afternoon I received a call from Mrs. C. asking if I had some time. Nancy's roommate was in the office with the message that Nancy very much needed to see usd in her dormitory room. Fortunately, I was free and accompanied them over to the dormitory. On the way, her roommate filled us in on the problem. Over the break Nancy had lost the baby. She was brought back to school lying in the back seat of the car, because she still did not feel well. But it was two days later and she did not want to miss any more school. However, she was still hemorrhaging and had to stay in bed.

When we arrived in the room, Nancy looked pale and weak, although she made an attempt to show some courage—though not so much to discourage sympathy. After the initial social amenities and consolations, we sat down beside the bed and she told us her story. She had gone to the doctor during spring vacation because she "felt that the baby was coming," even though it was much too early. The doctor soon realized that Nancy should be in the hospital; but before he could make arrangements the baby was born right there in the office. As the baby was emerging, the doctor reported that it was alive, and that it was probably about seven months along, but that there were "some problems." Alarmed, Nancy cried, "Oh, I want to see it; let me hold it." So the doctor put the baby in her arms while he called for an ambulance. Nancy, trembling and distraught, went on to describe and imitate the pitiable "death rattle" of the premature infant's labored attempts to breathe. After a few minutes, the baby died in her arms. Nancy was sobbing uncontrollably at this point, and somewhere in the telling of the story I had taken hold of her hand for comfort and support. During the most emotionally intense time, I realized that Mrs. C. in her empathy was also crying and not in very good shape herself. I also took one of her hands and for a while, as I attempted to be supportive to both women at the same time, I felt like an emotional lightning rod—conducting and stabilizing heavy current from all directions.

Eventually the catharsis ran its course and we were able to return to the present and the more mundane details of postpartum conditions.

After a while Mrs. C. and I left Nancy and took the opportunity to talk privately. We were concerned for Nancy's condition and had some uncertainty regarding the college's responsibility as well as liability. So we contacted the college health center and suggested that the nurse have Nancy brought over to be examined. This was done, and because of the continued bleeding Nancy was sent to the hospital for a gynocological consultation. The following day, the head nurse at the health center called us to tell us that she had an interesting report form the examining doctor: Nancy had not had a miscarriage. In fact, there had been no pregnancy. And he personally doubted if Nancy had ever even had intercourse.

The three subsequent counseling sessions that I had with Nancy were, needless to say, marked by confusion and embarrassment on her part. Initially, I attempted, as gently as possible, to relate to her the details of the hospital report, without recriminations or moralizing. Nevertheless, when you are forced to confront an elaborate fantasy with the uncompromising and harsh light of fact and truth, the inevitable result is shock. Frankly, I felt a little anxiety beforehand as I wondered if her hysterical personality was too fragile to handle this necessary confrontation. But I had to take the chance—relying on the close and trusting relationship that had been established. As it turned out, the session went about as well as could be expected. Naturally, there were some tears, but I did not allow them to be manipulative. As we talked, several times she interrupted the train of thought with the emotional exclamation, "I'm so ashamed; I don't belive I deceived the two of you that way—after all you've done for me. I don't believe I did that."

Once the fact of the false pregnancy was accepted, it was surprisingly easy to get to the bottom of the mystery. Nancy had no intention of deceiving her friends at school. We had merely got caught in the plot because we were involved in her life. The problem had begun in the first semester, when the boyfriend began to talk of breaking off the relationship. To prevent this from happening, Nancy had resorted to a frequent device for holding on to a man—she claimed she was pregnant. And because a blatant lie would conflict with her conservative moral upbringing, her unconscious mind created a condition that allowed her to believe it.

At the end of our conversation she was still saying, with sincere embarrassment, "I don't believe I did that." The confusion was as evident as the shame. It was as if a devious twin sister had pulled off this caper and let Nancy to suffer the consequences. But there was no twin sister, and to me it was a dramatic illustration of the close relationship between common "conversion" hysteria and the more extreme phenomenon of multiple personality. This woman did not go so far as to develop a different personality, with a different name, who took control over her life, but it came pretty close. I was able to arrange only one more session with Nancy that spring before the school year ended and she graduated. I believe that she realized, as well as I did, that there was more work to do. But year-end schoolwork was a handy rationalization for her avoidance of any more attention to the incident. Her nature desire was to forget that the whole thing ever happened. With her capacity for repression, that probably had not been too difficult. I continued to receive a Christmas card from her for several years, with newsy updates on her life. And things seemed to be going all right. Nevertheless, I would not have have been surprised to answer the telephone some evening and hear that familiar, clear soprano voice say, "Hello, Mr. Mac, this is **Jane**."

QUESTIONS FOR DISCUSSION

1. Do you understand, and can you explain, the difference between hysterical ailments and the psychosomatic symptoms resulting from anxiety?
2. Can you think of occasions when that "little kid" in your subconscious has tried to convince you that you are "too sick" to do something today? How do you handle these situations?
3. Do you think that Nancy's lifelong blindness had anything to do with her selection of a physical condition to resolve a problem?

Chapter
7

Alcohol Abuse
A Chemical Escape

MIKE S.: HAPPINESS IS BEING NUMB

Introduction

What do you really know about all of the effects of drinking alcohol? Of course, you have been confronted with questions like this since you were in junior high school—in the form of posters and lectures with boring statistics, along with warnings from every kind of authority figure. But how much attention did you pay? How often did you turn it off, thinking, "That doesn't apply to me"? Well, this reading is part of an important course that is part of your education. It is time to pay some serious objective attention. It may save your life, or at least preserve your precious right to have a choice of options available for your future, and to more fully realize your potential as a person.

Consider some of your most important personal needs:

1. You want to stay alive long enough to fulfill your important life plans. Thus, you certainly do not want to be part of these numbers: Roughly 100,000 Americans die every year as a direct result of inappropriate drinking of alcohol. Death may come from the failure of vital organs, such as the heart or liver or brain; or it may be caused by accidents in automobiles, boats, or airplanes, or from drowning, or falling out of upper-story windows. Seventy-five percent of automobile accidents and half of all automobile fatalities result from drunken driving. Almost all teenage automobile accident fatalities at night involve alcohol. One-quarter of all suicides are alcohol abusers. The immune system is adversely affected by alcohol. One scientist speculated that if it were not for alcoholics, we probably would have eliminated tuberculosis in America a long time ago. The bottom line is that people who drink alcohol unwisely will die early, one way or another.

2. You want to complete your education and go on to a successful career. Alcohol severely interferes with the learning process. (So do marijuana and most other drugs.) The brain cannot consolidate new material when it is trying to function in an alcohol environment. Alcohol is responsible for a very high percentage of student withdrawals from school for destructive or anti-social behavior or for academic failure. Given its impact on the learning process, it is an irony that alcohol is so popular with college students.

3. You want to become a mature and independent adult. Alcohol has a serious arresting effect on normal biological maturation. This is particularly true of emotional and sexual function. It is a typical and uncomfortable empathic experience to watch middle-aged alcoholic acquaintances as they struggle with withdrawal from alcohol dependence, suffer the intense pain of adolescent emotions that never had the opportunity to mature. Potential mothers must familiarize themselves with one of the most dramatic examples of this effect on maturation—the symptoms of fetal alcohol syndrome, which results from irresponsible drinking of alcohol when pregnant. Two of the characteristics that distinguish an adult from a child are controlled and stabilized emotional reactions and the ability to make clear and reasoned judgments and decisions. Excessive use of alcohol deprives one of both of these abilities.

4. You probably anticipate having a home and family someday. Alcohol abusers make terrible spouses and parents. One-quarter of American families have a drinking problem in the home. These are invariably badly disrupted homes. Forty percent of family court cases involve alcohol abuse. One-third of violence between mates, married or otherwise, results from drinking. One-third of child-molesting incidents involve alcohol. One-half of the country's homeless are alcoholics. The painful psychological scars from growing up with an alcoholic parent may last a lifetime.

When we take an objective look at the depressing facts about the effects of alcohol on human functioning, we have to inquire why in the world we drink it at all. Even worse, why is alcohol such a common, even dominant feature of our social and private lives? The answer, obviously, is that not all of its effects are undesirable. Some of alcohol's effects are so desirable that they override, even make us choose to ignore, the long-range negative consequences. What short-range effects could possibly be more important than the long-range consequences of early death or a messed-up life? The answer to this question evolves from the fact that alcohol is a psychoactive drug; that is, it affects the way the brain functions. Primarily and generally, alcohol acts as a central nervous system depressant. It acts differently on different parts of the brain, and differently in different people's brains. Much of the cause of this difference in the way people react to alcohol is inherited. But in general it slows down the brain and makes various of its functions sluggish and less efficient. With excessive amounts of alcohol, the brain is shut down to the point of unconsciousness or death.

The desirable psychoactive effects of alcohol are at least threefold. First, alcohol inhibits response from the punishment center in the brain, meaning that one is less able to experience feelings such as fear, anxiety, guilt, etc. This is a very desirable effect for most people and is the primary reinforcer for continued use of the drug. When people say, "Alcohol makes me feel good," for the most part they are really saying that alcohol keeps them from feeling bad. It is a cheap, legal, nonprescription tranquilizer. This partly explains its popularity as a social lubricant. With a little alcohol in us, we are less self-conscious and less inhibited or anxious about what other people are thinking. All of a sudden one becomes a great conversationalist, or dancer, or singer, or lover—at least one thinks so. A second desirable effect is to prevent withdrawal symptoms. For those people inherently predisposed to become physically dependent on the drug—in other words, addicted—the physical and psychological effects of abstaining from drinking alcohol are very unpleasant and cannot be tolerated for very long. The third desirable effect results from the fact that many brains are able to convert alcohol into an instant and efficient form of fuel, in place of sugar. Because alcohol passes directly from the stomach into the bloodstream and within a short time circulates to all organs, the conversion happens very quickly. This energizing effect probably accounts for the confusing impression that alcohol can act like a stimulant. Unlike normal people, most alcoholics actually perform more efficiently with a certain blood alcohol level than when they are sober, because their systems have become so accustomed to using alcohol as a fuel.

But why do we start drinking it in the first place? After all, there would be no opportunity to become psychologically or physically dependent on a drug if we never started using it. The same could be said for the widespread habit of smoking cigarettes to ingest nicotine, another poison. Again, because the behavior is so illogical and detrimental to our well-being, the forces at work must be powerful ones. This is a question of great concern for our society, because with each passing decade our children are beginning to experiment with and use alcohol (and other drugs) at ever younger ages. The result is the increased probability of becoming dependent on these substances, and therefore, an increase in the number of ruined lives, the amount of wasted human potential, and at the very least, a general decrease in the quality of adjustment.

There are many reasons why a person drinks, and certainly as many reasons why a young person would begin to drink. Therefore, we can discuss only in general terms the reasons that have been uncovered by social research. The foremost of these most likely is social acceptance—conformity to peer group behavior and pressure. Doing "what everybody's doing" is a powerful teenage motivation. Drinking is one of the many ways to express adolescent rebellion—experimenting with the forbidden. But how forbidden is it? Drinking often starts as part of social custom, ritual, or ceremony in the home. Drinking is likely to be part of self-concept exploration and enhancement. It can make a young person feel more grown up, mature, and sophisticated. It may allow the young person to emulate or imitate someone he or she admires. In this respect, advertisers and the mass media do not help at all. One of the most difficult challenges for adolescents these days is to make a well-reasoned and honest personal decision about whether or not to drink alcohol. And if they do, how much, under what circumstances, and for what reasons. It requires a great deal of courage and foresight to make a decision about what is best in the long run.

Any discussion of the problems associated with alcohol abuse must, of necessity, deal eventually with the much used terms "alcoholism" and "alcoholic." What is alcoholism? What is an alcoholic? They are troublesome terms to use accurately and correctly. These words do not communicate consistent meanings. There continues to be disagreement over definitions and the different perspectives among the experts. The term "alcoholic" evokes very negative attitudes and much social stigma in the vocabularies of most societies. Yet the drinking of alcohol is an accepted part of social custom in almost all cultures. The difficulty arises in the attempt to distinguish an alcoholic drinker from a nonalcoholic drinker. The definition used by Alcoholics Anonymous is a popular and respected one. This organization refers to an alcoholic as a person who is "powerless" to control his or her drinking of alcohol. As a result, the person's life has become unmanageable, resulting in serious problems with personal relations, health, finances, employment, and quite possibly the law. The criterion of "powerlessness" is an attractive one, as it implies loss of personal control and *addiction*. This is an important difference. The focus on problems resulting from drinking is a good idea, but it is not helpful in distinguishing an alcoholic from other drinkers. Anyone who drinks to the point of abuse, addict or not, is assuredly going to have problems with some aspect of his or her life.

The medical profession now refers to alcoholism as a disease and focuses on physiological and psychological symptoms. The disease concept has been helpful to the law in helping society to decide how to handle alcoholic behavior. For example, today the alcoholic is less likely to be put in jail, except for protective custody. It has begun to turn societal attitudes away from ideas such as "moral weakness" and "criminal irresponsibility" in reference to alcoholics. It has finally moved psychiatry away from the long-standing, firmly entrenched position that alcoholism is basically a mental illness. It has also helped relieve the alcoholic of some of the guilt over his or her condition. These are all positive changes. However, the question remains, is the disease concept valid? Unfortunately, it merely defines an ambiguous term with another ambiguous term. It is certain that abuse of alcohol can *cause* diseased conditions of virtually any organ in the body. But calling alcoholism a disease in itself is still not free from debate.

The frustrating fact is that there are very few dependable consistencies in the effects on different people of drinking alcohol. If we consider two individuals who have drunk approximately the same amount of alcohol, with the same frequency, for the same number of years, one may develop serious liver disease and one may not. One may have episodes of "blackout"; the other may not. One may develop problems from drinking fairly early; the other may cruise along for many years before developing serious problems. If both were told by a doctor, "You have to stop drinking immediately or you will be dead in a year," one may stop drinking with little difficulty, and the other may find it impossible without a great deal of help. The difference is that one is physically dependent and the other is not. One is an addict—and that is probably the crucial difference. The best simple definition of an alcoholic is an alcohol addict.

The evidence is finally fairly clear, after many years—generations—of faulty assumptions and disagreements. Some people are genetically predisposed to differential reactions to alcohol, and one of these is to addiction. This individual, pathological, physiological reaction to alcohol is called alcoholism. It is irreversibly progressive with continued use. It involves powerful physical addiction and psychological obsession with drinking. For alcoholics, perhaps the most dramatic reaction is loss of voluntary control of their drinking. For the alcoholic, life becomes a continuous preoccupation with maintaining the precise blood alcohol level in order to avoid withdrawal symptoms from drinking too little, and the personal disasters and public attention from drinking too much. Eventually, the bottle of alcohol becomes the addict's best friend—and finally, his or her only friend.

In the latter stages of this progressive diseased condition, the alcoholic manifests the psychological symptoms that give dramatic testimony to the effects of prolonged alcohol use on the brain: There is a bizarre distorted perception of reality, with delusional fantasies, grandiose unrealistic thinking, and paranoid fears. There is a stubborn denial of the truth about one's drinking, with elaborate rationalization. Judgment is seriously impaired, learning and memory are seriously impaired, possibly with blackouts—where the "video recorder" of the brain is turned off for periods of time. There is regressive immaturity as well as retarding and arresting of maturation. The emotional system is an unqualified mess with intense feelings of anxiety, fear, guilt, and bouts of depression. There is low frustration tolerance, with flaring, angry aggression. Finally, there is a settling into drunken isolation with pervasive self-hate. Early in my career, my concept of a continuum of quality of self-concept had, at the bottom end of the range, a condition typified by the statement, "I'm a zero." Later experiences with alcoholic friends and clients caused me to adjust the bottom end of the range down a notch to a state represented by, "I am a worthless and disgusting person." This represents a formidable challenge to sympathetic friends and relatives, as well as professional counselors. The one encouraging basis for hope or optimism is that most of these symptoms improve dramatically with sobriety. This is testimony for the position, now verified by scientific research, that psychopathology is not the cause of abusive drinking, but rather a symptom of it. An alcoholic drinks because he or she is an alcoholic.

The Case of Mike S.

Thinking back over the years to his childhood as we talked in my college office one afternoon, Mike could still clearly remember his first taste of beer. Even though the bitter taste made him wince and the foam made his nose crinkle, he smiled because this was the first time he had been allowed to share in the evening drinking. For a long time he had been his father's "go for." During his father's evening-long drinking sessions he'd say things like, "Go get me a beer, Mikey." "Thank you, Mikey, that's a good boy." Little Mike had willingly run these errands. It was one of the few ways to get attention or praise from his dad during those hours when he was totally focused on getting mellow and reading his newspaper or watching television. But until this particular evening, Mike's begging, "Can I have a sip, Daddy, can I have a sip?" had always been refused. It was one of the father's ways of denying that his drinking was having any effect on the family. No one could accuse him of being a bad influence on his children. It was Jim, Mike's older brother, who finally offered the boy a sip of his beer, mischievously expecting him to make an awful face. Jim himself was fairly young to be drinking a can of beer. But his father rationalized that "if he is only drinking at home, it will be all right." Actually, it was Jim's clandestine adventures with his friends outside the home that taught him how to appear to be unaffected by the beer, and to convince his father that it was okay.

Although the rule in the home continued to be "no more than a sip," it was only a matter of time before Mike began to feel that this was not fair. This was not being like everyone else and was for little kids, not grown-ups. By the summer that he was almost 12, he and a few friends had worked out a scheme that was like the secret games that his big brother, Jim, used to play. Every Saturday, each boy would sneak one or two beers out of their parents' refrigerators and meet at their secret place in the woods. This was fairly easy for Mike since Mr. S. purchased his beer one or two cases at a time and didn't bother to count cans until his supply began to run low. In their secret place the boys would have a ball—drinking beer, smoking cigarettes, and engaging in the rowdy, rough play of their favorite big, bad TV characters. In retrospect, Mike wondered how he and his friends managed never to fall out of the trees and break their necks. Two beers can really affect the judgment and coordination of a 12-year-old. But they never got seriously hurt, and they never got caught.

In the eighth grade, when Mike and his friends were 13, they began to experiment with "real booze." Thinking they were old hands at drinking beer, they wondered if hard stuff might be even more exciting. By this time there were girls in the gang of close friends, and they began to organize parties. It was easier for them to obtain permission to be out at night if there was a specific event at somebody's house. The boys began to steal whiskey and gin from their parents' house stocks and sneak it into the parties in thermos and soda bottles. Obtaining liquor was no more difficult a problem for Mike than getting beer. He had discovered that his mother kept a secret and secure supply of half-gallon jugs of gin hidden in a closet. He was at first startled by this discovery, but eventually began to figure it out. For a long time he had wondered why his mother never complained that his father did little but drink beer every evening until falling asleep about 9 o'clock. There seemed to be little shared home life or communication between them. Mike later realized that she did her own drinking, privately and secretly, in the daytime. There was an unspoken agreement: If you don't interfere with my system, I won't interfere with yours.

At their parties the teenagers designed what they considered to be very creative ways to play at their clandestine sophistication. At first they would sneak some gin or whiskey into the punch, and this system worked fairly well. Everyone would have a little and soon be feeling wonderful. With music playing to create the party mood and to muffle the occasional giggles or raised voices, they had a great time. To round out the imitation of their parents' parties, they added peanuts and snacks and even cigarettes to smoke—out the window, of course. However, this last detail of sophistication did not last long. They underestimated how far the smell of cigarette smoke would carry, and how long it would stay in the party room. Several parents cracked down and imposed stiffer house rules. Threatened with the loss of some of their best party places, the kids agreed among themselves to limit smoking to their secret places in the woods.

Inevitably, some of the boys eventually decided to try the greater excitement of drinking some hard stuff straight out of the bottle. This experiment was also short-lived. The kids were far too young to handle 100-proof liquor and quickly became rowdy and clumsy, and usually wound up being sick in the bathroom or out in the backyard. This behavior also threatened the loss of their party places and was outlawed by mutual agreement. Most of the boys privately had decided that the straight stuff tasted awful anyway. Their party drinking settled into mixing the alcohol with punch, orange juice, or tonic. Tonic was considered especially "cool"—the way the adults drank their gin.

Mike was often in a leadership role in the business of creative partying, partly because he had an extensive supply of exciting party stores from his big brother, Jim. This role also served to cover his quickly developing abnormal appetite for alcohol. His leadership evolved naturally as a result of the fact that Mike was beginning to mature physically a little earlier than his friends. He was perceived as being older. During those junior high school years, Mike's early maturation produced some additional benefits. He discovered that he could develop most athletic skills very quickly and easily. Because he was at least a year taller, stronger, and more coordinated than most of his friends, his participation was enlisted for any sports games. In fact, he was recruited for several of his school's athletic teams, and he was admirably productive in all of them. This was still the case when he was a freshman in high school, where he could compete even with the older boys. At the time, Mike had the world where he wanted it. He was admired and respected by his male and female peers, his teammates, his coaches, and his teachers. He was also blessed with an innate intelligence, which allowed him to maintain very good grades in school without an inconvenient amount of work.

By the spring of his freshman year in high school, at the grand old age of 14, Mike's drinking behavior began to show the first signs of going beyond social drinking and the first signs of alcohol dependency. During the week when his parents were not home, and when he was supposed to be doing homework, he began to sneak whiskey to his room. "Homework was so boring, and after a drink or two I began to feel that it was all right not to do it. I didn't feel guilty then. I could do what I wanted." At first this behavior was only occasional. But as time went on it increased to two or three times a week. He also began to experience restless sleep, hangovers, and stomachaches after these episodes. But those longer range punishments were easily forgotten under the enticements of immediate emotional relief and cravings for alcohol.

Unfortunately for Mike, this additional tapping of his mother's private cache finally aroused her suspicions and she shut off that source of supply with an angry lecture and locked up the liquor. But this was only a temporary setback to his system. He combined his allowance with money earned from odd jobs and used some older friends and his brother Jim as buyers, so he was usually able to obtain at least a pint bottle when he needed it. He was seldom lacking at least some emergency supply. And, in spite of these changes in his life, he still considered himself only a "weekend warrior" and a party drinker. The infamous alcoholic denial system was already forming, and doing its job of effectively clouding his perception of reality—at the age of 14.

As Mike's drinking increased in frequency, the inevitable consequences of abusing alcohol also began to show up as measurable negative changes in other parts of his life. As drinking increased in importance and his homework and athletic team practice proportionately decreased in importance, the problems began to appear. His teachers and the principal began to get on his case for cutting classes and being absent from school, or for coming to school smelling of liquor. The quality of his schoolwork was also slipping. His coach was becoming annoyed about his lack of commitment and enthusiasm and for missing practice.

Those of us who are concerned about the well-being of these youths who are in the process of destroying their lives by abusing psychoactive substances are apt to play the game of "in retrospect." We ask, why didn't any of the adults in Mike's life see the early warning signs and intercede more aggressively? But the reality of these situations is that people—like coaches and teachers—have far too many students to be responsible for to keep some of them from slipping through the cracks. Mike himself adds this explanation of the situation: "Remember, we were becoming pretty good liars and con artists by then. Also, at that time, my parents were too absorbed in their own problems and drinking to keep track of the details of mine. Besides, if anything was going to distract them it was the trail of disasters that my brother Jim was leaving behind him from his drunken escapades. He had already been kicked out of one college, had had several bad automobile accidents, been fired from several jobs, and had blown three or four good relationships. My parents had had to bring him home from police stations and hospitals any number of times after the vicious bloody brawls he got into in bars or at parties. All because of his drinking. And all before he was 20 years old."

Seeing what was happening to Jim's life did not deter Mike's own downslide during his remaining years of high school. It was predictable and depressing to watch. He was already hooked, and he had plenty of company on the way down. The effort he put into his schoolwork continued to decrease, virtually to zero. He had no motivation, no interest in much of anything except planning the next party. Oh yes, the parties continued. In fact, life became an almost continuous party. Whenever they had the ingredients, Mike and two or three friends would "kill" a two-liter bottle of Mountain Dew spiked with gin or vodka on the bus going to school in the morning. As his responsibility and dependability declined, he found it more difficult to get jobs for spending money. It became not unusual for Mike to resort to stealing liquor or the money to obtain it.

By his junior year there was no longer even any pretense at playing varsity sports. He decided that the practices were boring, took too much time, and there were too many rules. (Actually, he had been dropped from all of the teams and was no longer welcome at any team activities.) It is doubtful that he could have competed successfully by then anyway. His physical condition and coordination were already noticeably impaired by his drinking and lifestyle.

As juniors and seniors, Mike and his friends added a new, exciting variable to the fun and excitement of their parties—cars. In later years, in his "drunk-a-logues" at A.A. meetings, Mike told enough harrowing "car stories" to fill a book. Here are a few that he related to me:

> Our favorite car-party booze was called "jungle juice." In a gallon jug we would mix together—undiluted—anything we had except beer. That would make the mix foam up too much. We would pass the jug around and before long we were invincible, immortal, and fearless—cruising cool.
>
> One of our favorite driving games was "Dukes of Hazard." We would find a quiet piece of road that the police did not patrol very often, and we would try to get the car up to 100 MPH before we had to brake for a curve. One kid had rich parents, and he had a new souped-up Camaro. That car would do it easy. One night he drove it right into a lake going top speed—just like on TV. If it had been any deeper where the car sank, somebody would have drowned, we were so drunk. That kid totaled nine cars in three years. And the parents kept bailing him out. Stupid!
>
> My favorite game was "chicken." I'd drive down a road, straddling the center line, and scare the crap out of anybody coming along in the opposite direction. The most exciting thing was to come up in back of another car, suddenly, and then pass them over the double line on a hill. Some of them would almost hit the ditch, they were so startled. If another car had ever come over the top of the hill toward us, they never would have found all of the pieces—machine or bodies. I shudder at the thought of a kid of mine ever doing anything like that.
>
> One night we were parked beside the railroad tracks, quite a way from the road so we wouldn't be seen. It was after a party, but I was still sucking on a bottle. I was really blasted. All of a sudden I decided I was going to climb on top of one of those high signal holders that straddles the tracks. Then, I was going to jump down on top of the next train that came through and ride down to New York. They couldn't coax me down until my girlfriend started crying. I don't know why in the world I didn't fall off that thing.

Shortly after Mike turned 19, he "got lucky" and made a right turn off the highway to inevitable, hopeless, alcoholic hell. Recovering alcoholics and alcohol abuse counselors often speak of the important factor of "reaching bottom," before one is motivated to change his or her behavior and get sober. Mike did not hit bottom in the usual sense of destroyed career, or broken marriage, or alienated children, or the warning from a doctor that "at the present rate of deterioration you'll probably be dead in a year." But emotionally and psychologically he felt his face hit the rocks.

I believe that each of us, every few years, and without any particular conscious intent, stops paddling energetically against the current of social expectation and personal needs. We then turn around to look back and take inventory of what we have accomplished with our lives so far. It is difficult to say just what triggered Mike's personal inventory in his twentieth year. It may have been the stern and disgusted look on the judge's face as he revoked Mike's driver's license after his third D.W.I. accident and arrest. Or it may have been the recent ultimatum from his parents concerning "the conditions under which you can continue to live in this home." At any rate, when Mike turned around, what he saw was totally repulsive to him. He was intelligent enough to recognize a total waste of human potential. He was embarrassed to see a drunk running naked down the street—to the ridiculing amusement of onlookers, or to remember the several occasions when he woke up in bed with a strange woman—without any memory of how he got there. He was sickened by the deteriorated, abused body with its many scars and scabs. Each one was a reminder of the drunken brawls where he both delivered and received much pain. He was depressed by the lack of respect, or love and affection he engendered—no woman would stick with him anymore. And most depressing, he saw no growth or maturation. For one thing, he could not think of a single academic benefit from his last three years in school, although they had graduated him to get rid of him. Mike had reached that psychological state where the only self-descriptive word that fit was worthless.

Mike "got lucky," for several reasons. First, he was younger than most when he perceived that he was at the bottom and became motivated to turn his life around. He was also fortunate that he had not really become involved with a variety of addictive drugs, as most abusers have in recent years. He had stayed for the most part with alcohol, so that he had only one dependency to break free of. Third, he happened to have the right people around him when his moment of readiness occurred. As it happened, Mr. and Mrs. S. had recently celebrated two years of sobriety together, by virtue of consistent program work in both Alcoholics Anonymous (A.A.) and Alanon. So they knew what Mike was feeling, and they knew how to handle him. As parents, they had been learning to use the difficult principle of "tough love." This technique combines concern and support with firm confrontations of the drinker with the effects of his or her drinking—no more bailouts, no more denying. They had also been asking him some difficult questions about where he wanted his life to go, which may have had something to do with his self-inventory. The other people who had an important influence on Mike at this time were two friends who had recently gone through a similar enlightenment. At their invitation, Mike accompanied them to his first young people's A.A. meeting.

During much of the first year, Mike's involvement in the A.A. program remained tentative. His attendance was more dutiful than committed. He did not identify with the others to the extent that he was willing to admit or accept that he was an alcoholic. But he did manage to stay sober with his friends. By the time of his first anniversary of sobriety, Mike was noticeably healthier in body, mind, and self-respect. It was shortly thereafter that he began to understand the meaning of the twelve steps of A.A. The first two steps had particular personal meaning for him. He accepted the fact that he was helpless to control his drinking of alcohol. And the ambiguous "higher power" of the second step, in Mike's interpretation, referred to a forgiving and accepting God.

This awareness was a magic moment in Mike's life. It was the kind of insight or change of attitude event that we in the mental health field wish we could create at will. From this time on, the course of Mike's life achievements headed in a positive direction. He soon was assuming exemplary leadership roles in both A.A. and Alanon programs. He took a few part-time courses to test his readiness and then enrolled full time at a nearby junior college. Two years later he graduated with his associate degree, with honors. While he was there in college, he was a tremendous help to the counseling office in setting up a peer-counseling program for students having trouble with alcohol. He was also an invaluable help to me in setting up an on-campus Alanon group for students with alcohol problems in their families. He went on to earn two more college degrees, and now has a good job that allows his talents to grow. He also has a wife and child, and he continues to be active in the A.A. program— to protect his sobriety and his life.

Oh, about Jim: We buried him a few months ago. I'm not sure what finally caused Jim's death. Virtually every important organ in his body was damaged by alcohol. It was probably the failure of his liver; there wasn't much left of it anyway. And he was only about 35 years old.

QUESTIONS FOR DISCUSSION

1. How much do you really know about all of the effects of alcohol on your body and, more importantly, on your brain? How much do you want to know?
2. Do you pay attention to, or ignore, reports of results of new research on the effects of alcohol—especially the differential effects on women—when they appear in the news media?
3. Does Mike's drinking "career" in high school resemble that of any of your high school or college friends?
4. Have you ever tried to interfere, in a helpful way, with the self-harmful drinking behavior of a friend or relative? Did he or she pay any attention to your advice?
5. Is it useful or productive to suggest to a person that he or she might be an alcoholic? Why not?
6. Have you tried simply asking the person questions about how abuse of alcohol might be involved in some of his or her life problems?

7. Is there a possibility that alcohol, and/or other drugs, might be the cause of some of your life problems?
8. How much do you know about organizations such as A.A. or Alanon that can be helpful with alcohol abuse problems?
9. What are some of the ways that abuse of alcohol (and other drugs) can interfere with the needs, goals, or life tasks of a high school or college student?

Chapter
8

Other Substance Abuse: Cocaine

What Does Up Must Come Down, Down, Down

JOHN E.: HOW HIGH THIS GUY

Introduction

Chapter 7 introduced you to the adjustment problem of psychoactive substance abuse and dealt thoroughly with the country's biggest drug problem, alcohol. What do we discuss next? My original plan for the book was to tag onto the end of Chapter 7 a brief discussion of marijuana abuse, as it was long considered to be our second biggest drug abuse problems. However, alarming developments in recent years have persuaded me to change this plan. Cocaine has so rapidly and dramatically become the drug of choice for so many people that now you seldom hear about marijuana. Although people are still using and abusing "pot," it has been completely overshadowed in the media by government efforts, at all levels, to control the cocaine problem. It has reached epidemic proportions. Thus, we now think cocaine abuse deserves an entire chapter.

Why did cocaine suddenly become so newsworthy? Is it a new drug? What do you know about cocaine? Do you consider it a potential threat to your well-being?

Cocaine has become newsworthy for several reasons. Suddenly, well-known, healthy people (in particular, famous athletes) began dropping dead from overdoses of cocaine. Within a short period of time there was a rapid increase in the number of people of all ages becoming psychologically dependent upon and addicted to the substance—with all of the criminal activity and social problems that accompany such a phenomenon. "Coke," "toot," "blow," "snow," "snort," "C," "crack," "rock"—by whatever nickname it was called on the street, it had become the rage. It had also become a critically serious threat to the psychological and physical health of millions of people. When society is threatened by an enemy of this dimension, it demands that we learn all that we can about this enemy, so as to mobilize the best defenses we can.

A History of Cocaine

Cocaine is not, by any means, a new drug. It is a substance extracted from the leaves of the coca plant, which grows naturally in the valleys of the Andes mountains of South America. Native Indians of these regions have cultivated the plant and chewed its leaves for their psychoactive and medicinal effects for hundreds of years.

The most important chemical substance in the leaves of the coca plant is cocaine, which was first isolated and named in 1859. In the late 1800s cocaine, as an ingredient in various drinks, "tonics," and patent "medicines," became increasingly popular in the United States and in Europe. The most notable of these, of course, was Coca-Cola. Once the ability of cocaine to cause dependency and other ill effects became well known, a swelling of public concern resulted in the passage of the Harrison Act in 1914. Since that time, cocaine has been a controlled, illegal drug in the United States for all nonmedical use.

Predictably, making the drug illegal only shifted its merchandising to the black market. Because cocaine was a relatively expensive drug, this black market grew fairly slowly. But the growth was steady as cocaine became an increasingly popular recreational drug among the well-to-do. At first, cocaine was primarily used in its white powder form, cocaine hydrochloride. Then in the 1970s, there was a rapid increase in the use of cocaine due to a number of factors: a widespread general increase in psychoactive drug use, a general increase in affluence, an increased supply of cocaine in this country—with the resulting decrease in cost—and the appearance of a new form of coke called "free-base cocaine," which could be smoked for a faster, more intense experience.

Today there is an incredibly large, illegal market for all forms of cocaine. And because of the clandestine nature of the use and distribution of the drug, all efforts to accurately estimate the size of the present market have been frustrated. However, even conservative estimates put the number of cocaine users in the tens of millions. It is the focus of intense government drug control efforts and complicated international negotiations.

Cocaine's Psychoactive Properties

To understand the great popularity of cocaine, we must take a look at how it acts upon the nervous system and, in particular, the brain. Cocaine's psychoactive properties are directly opposite those of alcohol and the other depressants. It is a powerful central nervous system (CNS) stimulant. (Cocaine, incidentally, is different from other psychoactive drugs in that it has two additional unique properties. It is a local anesthetic, which decreases the pain sensitivity of nerve endings; and a vasoconstrictor, which decreases bleeding. It continues to be used legally for these properties in surgery on the eyes or nose.)

As a CNS stimulant, cocaine excites and speeds up all readiness responses. A person is quickly aroused, excited, alert, and displays all the other responses natural to an increase in the neurotransmitter norepinephrine. It imitates the human response to threat, competition, or stress. More important for our understanding of the desirable effects of cocaine is the increase in levels of the neurotransmitter dopamine in the brain. This produces a dramatic rise in euphoria, feelings of well-being and self-confidence, an artificial sense of being in control, sexual excitement, optimism, and the general ability to experience pleasure. All of this seems wonderful and very desirable. Everyone can be your friend. You can accomplish anything.

An additionally attractive characteristic that is appreciated by the "I want to feel better right now" mentality of the drug user is that cocaine's effects happen quickly—almost instantly in some cases. As a final bonus, unlike other recreational drugs cocaine gives no feeling of being drugged. For the person suffering the unpleasant feelings of anxiety, threat, guilt, remorse, insecurity, or depression, the instant relief of cocaine is a powerful attraction, especially if he or she is not very experienced or successful in coping with these feelings in more integrative ways.

Forms of Cocaine

Cocaine is used, for the most part, in two forms. As already mentioned, the older, more common form is cocaine hydrochloride—the familiar white powder. The chemicals in this powder are absorbed readily through the membranes of most of the body's external openings, but particularly the nose and mouth. The most popular way of ingesting cocaine in this form is to sniff or "snort" it into the nose. Within a few minutes, the chemical is in the bloodstream and flowing to the brain, producing that desirable euphoric high. Because cocaine hydrochloride can be dissolved in water, this solution can be injected directly into the bloodstream for an even faster, more intense "slam" effect.

The other form of cocaine is the cause of the extremely rapid increase in craze usage of the drug in recent years. Powdered cocaine can be chemically modified or "freebased" into a crystalline or "rock" form that carries the street name "crack." Freebase cocaine is not water soluble, but it does melt at a lower temperature and thus can be smoked. Because of the efficiency of the lungs at releasing gaseous chemicals quickly into the bloodstream, smoking crack produces an intense rush of stimulation and euphoria within seconds. Because an effective dose of crack can be obtained at a much lower cost, it has become increasingly popular and widely used at all levels of society. It has also become one of the hottest items on the criminal black market.

Cocaine has one more significant psychoactive property not mentioned earlier. Its desirable effects are very short-lived relative to other psychoactive drugs. The effects seldom last more than 30 minutes. Herein lies a significant part of cocaine's potential for abuse and threat to one's physical and psychological well-being.

Cocaine's Potential for Harm

Physical   Certainly first is the fact that you can die from using cocaine. Amounts of the stimulant reaching the brain can rise so quickly as to cause seizures, with loss of the brain's ability to regulate vital life functions. Strokes can also happen, with resulting paralysis of parts of the body. Cocaine's effects on the heart can be equally dangerous. Its action of increasing heart rate, and at the same time constricting blood vessels carrying oxygen to the heart muscle, may cause chest pains or a heart attack. This makes it particularly dangerous for people with existing heart problems or high blood pressure. In addition to making the heartbeat more rapid, cocaine may also produce an irregular heartbeat (arrhythmia), which can be life threatening.

As is the case with most drugs, cocaine can cause a number of complications to pregnancy. Because an unborn fetus shares its mother's blood supply, it is subject to all of the effects of cocaine on the mother. In addition, other hazards include spontaneous abortion, premature death, physical deformities, or any of the effects of a decreased flow of blood to the unborn child, particularly to its brain.

Worth mentioning are a number of other, less serious, physical consequences of using cocaine. Sniffing coke into the nose can cause nosebleeds or damage to the septum in the nose. Smoking crack, at the least, causes bronchitis and hoarseness, but may also damage the lungs.

Psychological   As students of psychology, we are particularly concerned with the ways that this substance can affect our thinking and feeling and the way we manage our lives. It is in these areas that cocaine's natural properties make it one of the most insidious and dangerous drugs.

The reason that the wonderfully pleasant but artificial feelings of euphoria, well-being, and self-confidence do not last very long is that the brain's reaction to restore its own equilibrium is, in this case, very effective and efficient. Within 30 minutes the effects are reversed and, as is often the case, overcompensated for. What goes up must come down, down, down! Replacing happiness are feelings of fatigue, depression, irritability, pessimism, anxiety, and sometimes even thoughts of suicide. Coming down from a cocaine high can be very unpleasant, and reality seems worse than it was before. The brain no longer functions normally in many ways. Overstimulation causes it to become confused. The focus of attention constantly flits from one thing to another. Perception of reality becomes distorted, even bizarre. The whole nervous system is on edge. The emotions are disrupted. You feel anxious, worried, insecure. Stressful situations can seem even more intimidating than usual.

But most of this unpleasantness is easily and quickly remedied—by snorting another line or smoking another hit on the pipe. It is frighteningly easy for these cycles to become habits, then compulsions. With continued repetitions the crash-downs become worse. The bad feelings are more awful. The distorted perceptions can approach psychotic seriousness. The abuser may come to feel paranoid about people—suspicious of their motives. "They" seem to be out to get you, to steal some of your precious supply, or to get you in trouble. Police, teachers, co-workers, bosses, or others in authority are particularly suspect.

With continued use cycles, the need to get rid of the bad feelings and get the good feelings back can become a powerful, even irresistible craving, and control is gradually lost. This is the terrible trap of cocaine. The irresistible cravings become a psychological addiction. The craving becomes so powerful it supersedes all other needs. Everything else becomes unimportant and neglected: schoolwork, the job, home, responsibilities; relationships, the sensible and responsible management of money. The high cost of coke quickly uses up savings and throws one into debt; all the threats to health are ignored; even food and nutrition become unimportant.

The significance for the student here is obvious. Work assignments, deadlines, and tests may be ignored. Relationships may be destroyed. Money for college expenses may be blown on cocaine. This may be the fastest way known to substance-abuse your way out of school or your job.

With this general information in mind, let us consider a real-life story.

The Case of John E.

At one point in John E.'s senior year in high school, during one of his many introspective moments, he got to thinking that he couldn't even remember when or if he had ever really been satisfied with himself. He was probably a normal high school kid. But, in his own eyes, it was difficult to think of any particular personal attribute about which he could say, "I'm okay." He had a fair number of friends, or at least kids he could hang around with. But he didn't feel really close to any of them. He often felt ill at ease and awkward when trying to carry on a conversation—especially with most of the girls. As a result, he spent a lot of time alone, although he didn't particularly enjoy that either. He didn't have any trouble understanding what was going on in his classes, so he didn't feel dumb. But high school for the most part was boring to him. He did only as well as he had to, to keep his parents and teachers off his back. He usually did his assignments at the last minute, and they were usually no better or worse than average. But as long as this system worked he used it. He wasn't getting a great deal out of school, but he also didn't have to spend much time studying. He played sports with the other boys, but he had no interest in being a jock and would rather talk a good game when he could get away with it. This involved no commitment, no moments of testing or proving himself.

John didn't even like his name. It annoyed him a little that the girls often called him Johnny. He never expressed these feelings to any of them, but the nickname was too much like the more formal John E. that his mother and some of his relatives used to distinguish him from his father. His father had the same first name but a different middle initial.

What he *did* like about his school years and the summers were the parties. These were the only times that he felt comfortable and relaxed. It seemed that most of his life consisted of being and doing what everyone else—either his parents, his teachers, or his peers—expected him to be and do. There never seemed to be opportunity to negotiate these expectations. It was so rare that anyone asked, "What do you want, John?" that he didn't even know. But, at the parties, sometimes there was beer, or spiked punch, or even some marijuana. It didn't matter; they all produced the magic effect of relaxing him. With just a little, you could forget the pressures or just not care.

As he progressed through high school, a life-style became fairly well established. Last-minute production of the required work and a series of part-time jobs maintained the appearance of responsibility, although being responsible was not yet a high priority to him. He came increasingly to identify with the party people, because they knew how to get feeling good and be cool. However, none of them had the insight at this time to realize that these feelings were entirely artificial. They were aware that other groups of kids were into "coke" and "crack" and other stronger drugs. But John's crowd did not have the money for that sort of recreation. Besides, those other kids were "drug users," and being a "druggie" was different.

All in all, the high school years were not bad for John. There were occasional feelings of emptiness where there ought to have been a sense of bonding or of close meaningful relationships. And he was missing any sense of accomplishment or purposefulness. But he had found a reliable system for ignoring these things and relieving the tensions of unfulfilled needs. Alcohol and pot were effective and convenient medicines.

However, when the time came to think seriously about college and applications, the coasting life-style was brought to an abrupt end. His parents—primarily his father—were disturbed and angry to realize that John's cumulative high school grades were below average. They had not been low enough to attract much attention earlier but were much too low for him even to consider applying to one of the good schools to which John's father wanted him to go. In an angry, loud lecture, Mr. E. expressed his disappointment with John's wasted high school years and made it clear that he expected his son to go to college and to be successful. The point was not debatable; there was no alternative, unless John wanted to support himself with an unskilled job.

Under the circumstances, the only route into an "acceptable" college was to detour through the community college system, where entrance requirements were more lenient and where he would have an opportunity to "get his act together." John's two years in a state community college certainly brought about some changes. Operating under the new motivation of fear, he actually learned to do some hard academic work, or at least devote more of his time to it than he had before. Also, under the influence of some professors he liked and some more mature students in his classes, he actually developed some ambition, curiosity, and personal independence. Unfortunately, the habits and skills that John had developed in high school were not abandoned totally, only modified. While he learned how to work hard, often it was still at the last minute and under the gun of deadlines. He continued to deal with stress and tension in the same way—by partying. He also learned to party harder. It was easier to find a hard-drinking crowd in college, especially with the decreased need for secrecy.

After two years, however, it appeared that John's junior college period was a success. He acquired academic and verbal skills sufficient to earn his associate degree, with a grade point average that was well above average. He also developed some social assertiveness and self-confidence. He learned how to work to a successful outcome. He developed a hard-driving, success-oriented personality and life-style, which his father admired. He was accepted by a university that was satisfactory to both his parents and himself, qualified for some scholarship and loan assistance, and received a commitment from his father to supply more financial assistance.

The summer between John's second and third years of college could be described as a prolonged three-month celebration. He frequently found himself singing a line from some song, which went: "We're on our way . . . " He couldn't remember the rest. But these were the words that gave vocal expression to his new confidence. His away-from-home summer job provided the opportunity to earn some decent money, but also left plenty of off-hours time for some great partying with other young people at the same resort.

Two significant events occurred during that summer. We might already be aware that John's "success story" of the past two years was, at this point, only a fragile house of cards. It would take little to change the direction from success to failure. The first of these events was John's chance meeting, at one of the parties, with an attractive girl who immediately aroused more than the usual interest on his part. As a result of numerous after-party adventures in the past, John had acquired some romantic and sexual skills and a fair amount of experience. He had never taken any of these relationships very seriously, and in fact had carefully avoided allowing any of them to become an emotional commitment. However, Jane was different. After only a couple of dates he realized he wanted to stay with her. Jane, for her part, was equally attracted to his winning (albeit alcohol-induced) glibness, charm, and self-confidence. For the first time in his life, John had a steady girlfriend. They were a couple for the remainder of the summer and on into the fall, after they reunited at the university in September. One of the early facilitators of conversation, at their first meeting, was the fact that she too would be a student at the university.

The second event of that summer was when one of the more affluent young men brought some cocaine to share at one of the parties. This was, surprisingly, John's first experience with a cocaine high, and he was delighted. "This is nice stuff; why haven't I tried it before?" There was one more opportunity for him to experience the pleasant effects of snorting cocaine that summer, and this time Jane was with him to share it. On both of these occasions he had already had a few drinks of alcohol, so that the effects were somewhat blurred. But, even though he was not yet aware of the full impact of a cocaine rush, the stage was set for events to come.

The first semester of his junior year at the university was more of an adjustment for John than the transition from high school to junior college had been. There was much more reading and more sophisticated understanding was required; the competition was, in general, more intense. Some of the classes were much larger, and the professors were more distant and less available. John quickly discovered that his old system wasn't going to work any more. The grades on his first tests and papers were much lower than they had been in the past. By mid-semester he was significantly behind in several classes, and was seriously concerned about whether he would pass three of them. He was also beginning to worry about what his parents would do if things did not improve by the time semester grades came out, and what would happen to his scholarship.

It was a comfort to have Jane for a dependable companion and friend. She was a more conscientious and competent student, and to some degree set a good example for him. But it began to depress him to realize that he could not give what he did not have. And he did not have the ability to meet these academic demands. He began to rely even more on his old medicines for cheering up and courage—alcohol and marijuana.

He began to drink and smoke more frequently during the week. He was disappointed that Jane now frequently refused to join him. He also was getting annoyed that, instead of being encouraging, she was beginning to chide him for his lack of responsibility. He began to feel forced into rationalizing the changes in his behavior. "Hey, pressures are rough. A person needs to relax once in a while. I'm not doing anything different from other people. I can handle it. It's all part of my plan. I'll come through; you'll see." Of course, it began to be "partly her fault" that he needed to drink more, because "she was letting him down and being a nag." But, in moments of honesty, he could see that his old system wasn't working. While a few beers and smoking a couple of joints had always been somewhat socially acceptable ways to relax the tensions, there was no denying that these drugs made him sloppy-headed and uncoordinated. He made bad judgments and mistakes. His perception of the world became different from the reality when he was sober. There was always the hours of sobering up and the hangovers to face, too. He was in that position where, once a pattern of psychological dependence on chemicals is established to relieve the daily tensions and anxieties, eventually there is a desire for something more and different. And for John it took only one good hit of cocaine to discover what the something more was.

The opportunity for this discovery was offered one Wednesday night, when one of John's dependable drinking buddies showed up with a small bag of white powder suggesting that "they try something different for a change." The timing was perfect. John had been feeling depressed and demoralized and close to being beaten by the workload, the deadlines, the fatigue, and his flagging motivation. John imitated his friend by making a couple of thin lines of the powder on a small mirror. Then he put one end of a short straw in his nostril and sniffed the lines of powder into his nose through the other end. John was almost overwhelmed by the reaction. The instant rush through his whole system was awesome. The total effect on his nervous system was like that of an orgasm. Unpleasant feelings were numbed and replaced by a warm sense of confidence. The delusion of being in control again was marvelous. Everything was okay and was going to stay that way. After a while he came to an inspired and obvious conclusion: Why struggle so hard for limited success when the illusion of success was so easy to come by. It was disappointing that the effects didn't last very long, however, but the friend had brought enough coke to keep them high for the night. He didn't realize it at the time, but the "friend" was setting up a new customer. Before long, John was hooked. He was going to be a winner and a hero again.

John didn't have enough money at that time of the year to pursue any large or consistent cocaine habit. But he did manage to scrounge enough cash, one way or another, to finance an occasional binge. And several of the occasions produced incredible feats of endurance and production, as far as schoolwork was concerned. He believed he had discovered the "jet fuel for success." Under the influence of cocaine highs he believed he could speed-read entire assignments. And he was able to write "brilliant, original" term papers at blinding speed. On one occasion he was concerned that if he worked any faster, his machine would begin to smoke. Unfortunately, the test scores that this system produced did not quite match his expectations. Parts of the "brilliant" papers were so incoherent that professors gave up trying to comprehend them. Nevertheless, he was for the first time getting work in on time. He managed to pass all of his courses—though just barely in some cases—and was able to continue on to the spring semester with only an academic warning.

The spring semester of John's junior year included some gradual but significant changes. He became less of a "party animal" and his use of all drugs, including alcohol, became more solitary. He had to find some rationalizations for these changes. But his medicines were now too important to him to risk having to share them. He was now more preoccupied with thinking about drugs and making careful plans to assure that an adequate supply was available when it was needed. This not infrequently involved "reassigning" some of his allowance and other money that was intended for necessary college expenses. It meant that he did not buy books that could be borrowed or obtained elsewhere. It often meant not buying food. And it meant "postponing" the payment of telephone bills and other charges that could be delayed. Although he was able to borrow money for a while, his personal credit dried up when his friends began to realize that they probably would never be paid back. Besides, his grandiose thinking was becoming so bizarre that it no longer could even be taken humorously, and they no longer believed much of anything he said.

Jane tried to stick it out with him for a while. She cared for him and cared about what was happening to him. But she gradually came to realize that there was less and less for her in the relationship. John never did seem capable of any real depth of affection or intimacy, and he became angry when she complained of this. She did not care to share in his excessive use of alcohol and cocaine, and she could not share in his get-high-and-work binges. She felt she was becoming much less important to him than his drugs—as was everything else in his life. Paradoxically, she was also becoming afraid of his paranoia and jealousy. He would unfairly accuse her of infidelity, and go into rages when he saw her with any other men. He would call her in the middle of the night to see what she was doing and become furious if she wouldn't get up and go out with him or let him come over. After a while she regretfully terminated the relationship for the sake of her own survival.

The departure of his best friend from his life was a painful blow for John and caused him to feel more alone than he ever had. But he adjusted to the situation in the same way he now handled all pain and stress—plenty of booze and coke, when he could get it. He also rationalized that "he was really better off without her" and "she was getting to be a drag anyway."

John barely squeaked through the spring semester of that junior year by following his established system of isolated drug binges and flurries of frenzied work. However, the situation was more precarious. The academic dean's office put him on probation for the beginning of the following year. If he could not bring his grade point average up to a level where graduation was more assured, he would be withdrawn. He wasn't exactly in good standing with the office of the Dean of Student Life either. He had accumulated warning letters in his file for unacceptable social behavior involving being drunk and disorderly, and for harassment.

John returned to his old job at the resort that summer, hoping for a break from the stressful roller-coaster ride of stress and ecstasy that college life had become. In sober moments during those summer months, when he missed the fun he had had with Jane the summer before, he began to experience some insights into the failure of the relationship. The insights were probably triggered by his recalling some of her complaints about his not letting her feel close to him or share real intimacy. He realized that this was not the first time that this had happened. He had dated other girls more than once, but had never let any of them get very close either. Perhaps the reason he had let her go without more resistance was that the cocaine-induced sense of well-being was a more than adequate substitute for real emotional intimacy. Cocaine was also a less complicated lover. But it was lonely between the artificial highs. Why couldn't he let people get close? He would describe his family as being close, but only to the extent of being loyal and having strong family identification. Although his parents had properly taken care of all of his needs as a boy, he couldn't remember ever being hugged, or being allowed to cry or to be afraid. The word that best described emotions in his home was "insulated." There were never displays of anger or affection. He had always had the impression that feelings would have complicated the arrangement. If we don't share or express feelings, then we don't deal with love. Not knowing if we are loved or lovable leaves a sizeable space in our self-concept, which can drive us to a continuous searching for ways to fill it.

Because the summer job was so much less stressful than school, John actually used less alcohol and cocaine than he did during the school year. Nevertheless, the periods of sobriety necessarily brought about a less distorted perception of reality. He could not help thinking about the miserable condition his life was in as he approached his 21st birthday and legal maturity. His academic career was a disaster. His social life was empty and artificial. His parents were disappointed in him, and he was no less disappointed in himself. Because these preoccupations were too depressing to endure for long, he would occasionally use some of his summer earnings to purchase a small supply of cocaine. By this time he had discovered "crack," the smokable crystalline form, and eagerly sought its powerful instant rush of relief from his depressions.

It was during one of these artificial highs that he had his "brilliant" and "original" idea. Unavoidably his biggest problem was money. His cocaine trips were using summer earnings that were supposed to be saved for college expenses. He had constantly been in financial trouble during the past year. His father had threatened that if John spent any more college expense money for unauthorized use, no matter what excuse John came up with, he was going to withhold further support. John's brilliant plan was to "cut out the middleman" and become a seller himself. According to this plan, he would buy a larger supply of cocaine on the wholesale market, sell it for twice what he paid, and make huge profits. As a bonus, the cocaine for his own use would be free. He even fantasized about being financially independent of his father or anyone else, and being able to get even with those who refused to lend him money the year before.

In the fall, John returned to school for the start of his senior year with a renewal of his old enthusiasm and dynamic ambition. He was going to "leave deep tracks in the road this year." More than once he might have been heard muttering to himself, "Watch my dust, baby, I'll be on top again before they even know what's happening." He did manage to make contact with a wholesale supplier of cocaine. At a highly secretive and somewhat scary meeting in the city with "this South American guy," he turned over his entire savings from the summer job for his first large stock of cocaine.

For a while the rest was easy, just as he had planned. By the simple device of undercutting the price of his old dealer, and by taking advantage of his knowledge of users on campus, he was able fairly quickly to acquire a list of 20 to 30 customers. By word of mouth, the referral list increased even more. By the end of September he had made several more quick trips into the city, buying bigger stocks of coke each time. At times, his pockets contained large amounts of money. His fortunes and his confidence were soaring like a Fourth of July rocket into the sky. He was a big man again.

But Fourth of July fireworks reach a peak of brilliance and power, then fizzle and burn out, and drift back to earth. And reality soon closed in on John and his plans. As he poured his time and energies into his new business venture, he almost totally neglected his academic responsibilities. Most of the first assignments were not due until several weeks into the semester. But he lost track of time and the dean began to receive periodic progress reports on him indicating tests failed or missed entirely, sporadic class attendance, and various work assignments not submitted to professors. In the first week of October, John received a serious warning letter from the dean reminding him that his academic probation status would be reviewed at mid-semester. He was also beginning to receive warnings from his dormitory director, the campus police, and the town police department, concerning rumored reports of his drug-dealing activities.

As familiar pressures and anxieties mounted, John slowly but steadily increased the number of his relief trips into his cocaine supply. He was aware that this was happening, but it was easy to rationalize since he now had so much on hand most of the time. Soon the "free" portion of his stock was gone before it was time to resupply, and he was dipping into the portion allocated for resale. As he snorted and smoked more of his profits, he had less money to restock; he began to turn away customers to assure enough supply for himself. The down times between highs became more and more intolerable. His anxiety and depression were awful, and his thoughts became paranoid. He was convinced that everyone was watching him, waiting to turn him in or steal his supply of cocaine or his money. He was so high most of the time that sleep, let alone any kind of relaxation, became impossible. His thinking became increasingly disorganized and flitted from one subject to another, with no logical connection. It frightened him that he could not control the rapid pounding of his heart, or his jitteryness, or what his mind was doing—he had thoughts about running away, and even about ending it all.

Near the end of October, John's paranoia received a dreadful reinforcement. Late one night, as he was returning from a delivery in a secluded part of the campus, he was suddenly confronted by his former dealer. After severely beating him he left John lying on the ground, half conscious and bleeding from the face, with the warning, "Get out of business in my territory or next time I'll use a knife."

John struggled back to his room, locked the door, and seldom came out of it again for nearly a week. He no longer needed any excuses to seek the relief of his white powder "medicine." All of his fears, anxieties, and suspicions were now justified. He reached a deep and profound bottom of the human condition during that week, during which he was fortunate he did not die from an overdose or the side effects of excessive cocaine use. I have often marvelled at how the body and brain can not only survive but recover from the effects of drug abuse, especially in cases like this. There were almost no breaks in John's desperate attempts to prevent the dreadful crashes into fear, anxiety, despair, and suicidal thoughts. The brain has an amazing capacity to compensate for the psychoactive effects of stimulants. It became more difficult for John to reach and maintain the highs. Even worse, the highs themselves took on a terrifying quality of their own. One cannot depress the accelerator pedal indefinitely to keep the motor running at high speed, without some compensating opportunities for rest, sleep, and restoration of fuel. Inevitably resources will become exhausted, and there will be a physical and mental burnout and a crash. Eventually, the prolonged overstimulation of his brain's ability to process information from his senses caused the normal distortions of perception to become hallucinations, and he lost his ability to control his contact with reality. His buzzed-up world became as terrifying as his depressions. He saw faces peering in the windows and through the cracks in the doors. He was convinced that sand fleas—from his summer job at the beach—had hidden in his luggage and were now crawling and hopping everywhere around him, in his bed, in his clothes, in his hair, and all over his skin. There were snakes in his closet and spiders in his dresser drawers, and in a box of crackers when he opened it. There was no escape from the torment.

Late at night on the fifth day of John's isolation, his piercing screams of terror and childlike crying aroused the other students on his floor. When the dorm director and campus police unlocked John's door, they found him curled in a chair, feet tucked up under him, and his arms and hands wrapped over his head in desperate self-protection. This pitiful frightened person was the same one who, a month earlier, was riding the top of the wave, with the illusion that he was in marvelous control of his destiny.

John was strapped to a stretcher with restraining belts and rushed to the detoxification unit of the hospital. Because the doctors were uncertain about the outcome of this case, an emergency call was made to his parents. If he survived, they would take him home from college for the last time.

Ironically, a letter from the dean's office was already lying in his college P.O. box. It stated that he had been expelled from the college for failure to meet the conditions of his academic probation, and for violations of college rules regarding use and distribution of illegal substances. One can only speculate how long it would be before John could even read this letter.

Because John's story is a composite case, it could have any one of several endings. His heart might fibrillate and he would die. His brain might go into seizure and he would die. A stroke might leave him paralyzed or incoherent for a long time. The consequences of heavy use of stimulants are unpredictable. He could be psychologically impaired for a short time, a long time, or forever. Or he could recover completely with good hospital care and with the long-term support of a twelve-step recovery program and of other recovering addicts and his family. He would need assistance in reexamining his life-style, his needs, and the nonintegrative habits he had developed for dealing with pressures and stress. Most important, he might be helped to a whole new assessment of his self-worth. I'll let you pick the ending.

QUESTIONS FOR DISCUSSION

1. What did you learn as a result of reading this chapter?
2. Do you now have a better understanding of what might become a new concept in the vocabulary of drug abuse—"psychological addiction"?
3. Does taking cocaine sound as though it might be a pleasant experience?

4. Did this story do anything to persuade you not to get involved with this dangerous drug?
5. What other arguments or ways can you think of to convince people not to experiment with cocaine?
6. If you were in charge of a drug awareness campaign in your school, what hazards of cocaine use and abuse would you give the most publicity?
7. Do you have an opinion regarding the probable long-term outcome for John?

Chapter
9

Eating Disorder: Anorexia

The Deadly Diet

JUNE S.: "YOU CAN'T BE TOO THIN"

Introduction

While sitting at lunch with several faculty colleagues a few months ago, I overheard one of my female colleagues state this bit of often quoted philosophy, "You can't be too thin or too rich." I had always considered this person to be an intelligent and sensible woman, so I had to check my assumption that she was being sarcastic or facetious. But from all indications she was serious. I thought, "What a pessimistic and depressing testimony on the tyranny of cultural norms!" I have become accustomed to the obsession of freshman college women with their diets and clothing fads. But, when more mature and intelligent women become that distracted from more important human values, then something is psychologically unhealthy with a society's value system. In my opinion, the villains are the media creators in Hollywood and the fashion magazine people, who present artificial and idealistic standards of beauty to be emulated.

The trend is given legitimacy and credibility by the medical professionals who insist that an alarming proportion of the American population is overweight to an unhealthy degree. They are, of course, correct. One merely has to return to this country after traveling in almost any other country to see immediately the contrast in body shapes. However, some of those who have heard the message seem to have been carried away. The medical view that slender is healthy and fat is unhealthy has become modified in social attitudes into thin is beautiful and fat is ugly. It has become a rare experience to talk to an American female who is not on some kind of diet. Of course, being diet and weight conscious has a healthy significance for one's long-range well-being. But becoming obsessed with thinness, without appropriate knowledge and information, is unhealthy and can be dangerous. The uncompromising social dictum "fat is ugly" also has negative implications for psychological adjustment. Building and maintaining a positive and comfortable self-image are difficult processes for most people in our complicated culture. It becomes nearly impossible, however, for millions of people who inherit metabolisms or physical conformations that are above the normal range for weight and build. It also complicates the already difficult adjustments that teenagers face in adolescence. Social science research indicates that most adolescent girls tend to have an initial negative perception of the heaviness in their hips and thighs as their bodies assume mature female proportions. If society reinforces this perception, then girls may be motivated to resist their natural development.

The epitome of this condition is a modern psychopathology that was virtually unknown a few generations ago—anorexia nervosa. Anorexia is a serious eating disorder that has attracted increasing attention and concern among medical and psychological professionals. The magnitude of the problem in terms of national statistics is difficult to estimate, partly because the young females who are affected are secretive about their behavior. The anorexia population is almost exclusively females in their middle to late teens (roughly 95 percent), although the illness not infrequently extends on into the twenties. The young women are usually first referred for medical treatment because of severe weight loss and refusal to eat normally. They are often subsequently hospitalized for treatment of malnutrition, to regain control of their intake of food, and for treatment of other difficult symptoms. These other symptoms are primarily psychological: anxiety, depression, an obsessive fear and revulsion of being fat, and a distorted and unrealistic perception of what their bodies look like. It is also common for their menstrual periods to become irregular or to stop entirely.

Anorexia is a difficult problem to treat. In spite of increasing sophistication of treatment, only about two-thirds of its victims are eventually cured. The remainder continue to be ill, and about 25 percent of the cases eventually die. It seems obvious that lack of cooperation by the patient is a large factor. Treatment now includes attacking the problem from all sides. First is a supervised restoring of proper nutritional intake—forced if necessary. To save their lives, the girls must be made to begin eating properly again. Systems of behavior modification are used to induce cooperative behavior by the patient. Finally, psychotherapy is used in three ways: individual, patient groups, and family groups.

As with all illnesses that are difficult and mysterious, attention becomes focused on the questions of *what causes* this problem, and *what can prevent* it from getting started in the first place. Although science is actively studying the problem, the present status of knowledge is best described as one of debate and speculation. This inevitably is the case when we are confronted with chicken-and-egg controversies over cause and effect and heredity versus environment. For example, in this case we have the questions: Do hormone imbalances trigger the distorted thinking and unhealthy behavior, or are abnormal hormone levels the result of the failure to eat properly? Are strong, disturbed emotions the result of abnormal brain chemistry or abnormal endocrine gland activity or environmental stresses?

Rather than dwell on questions we cannot answer at this time, let us inventory the facts that *are* known about anorexia and what they contribute to our understanding. The following are relatively consistent variables in the anorexia syndrome:

—Anorexia occurs almost exclusively among adolescent females in the middle and upper social classes.

—The girls tend to be intelligent, perfectionistic superachievers. They have high ideal self-images that they strive to live up to. Anorexia is often referred to as the "good-girl" syndrome.

—Anorexics have abnormal levels of some hormones, particularly the sex hormones. Also, it is typical for their menstruation to cease at some point during the illness, sometimes even before the pattern of weight loss.

—There is a strong emotional component, with anxiety, depression, and anger being the most common.

—There is an obsessive fear of being fat and a compulsion to avoid eating.

—The variable of *control* is consistently present. Most anorexics seem to be seeking some aspect of their lives over which they have complete control.

—Anorexics tend to perceive their mothers as too dominating or protective.

This list makes it possible to understand why current theorizing leans to the role environment plays in the disease. It is most commonly an American, upper-social-class problem. It is almost exclusively an adolescent female problem, although there are consistent personality variables. But, before we commit the scientific error of closing our minds to other possibilities, or condemning American values and families too harshly, we should keep this in mind: Millions of girls are subjected to the same social, family, and personal psychological pressures without developing anorexia nervosa. We must continue to search for what makes these girls different.

A fairly typical case history illustrates many of the points that we have been discussing about anorexia.

The Case of June S.

June's story is actually a composite of two stories. The original stories were written for me in the form of autobiographies, submitted as partial fulfillment of course requirements. At that time June was a 19-year-old sophomore, who was doing remarkably well after years of a harrowing struggle with anorexia. However, she still was working out residual questions regarding her self-concept, her feelings, her personal relationships, and her life goals. Writing the story was as helpful to her as it is to us, and serves as a guide to some overall understanding of this illness.

June S. grew up in a fairly typical middle-class community in a suburb of Philadelphia; her home and family were unpretentious, but economically secure. Her father was a middle-level business executive, and her mother also held a managerial position in business. Both parents had moderately strong, though not overbearing, personalities. They conveyed high expectations for themselves as well as their children, regarding schoolwork or any other responsibilities. By personal example they set a clear standard that mediocrity was not acceptable. "If it is worth doing at all, it is worth doing well." They were conservative, church-going people. Their home was family centered with obvious consideration and concern for each other's welfare. It seemed important to the children, or to the girls at least, to please their parents. June has one older brother and two younger sisters.

June's story begins in the fall of her freshman year of high school. Her clearest memories of that September focused on feelings of anxiety as she faced a new school with its challenges. She remembers also that this is the time her feelings of depression began, although the depression was probably related more to conditions at home than to those at school. It was then that her older brother, a senior in high school, was at his worst in a period of anti-social behavior that covered a span of several years. He was continually in trouble with the school administration and the police for drug use, drinking, speeding in his car, and truancy. His behavior created an uncomfortable amount of turmoil and tension in their home. It was a problem that no one seemed to be able to control. During the early weeks of that school year, June worried continually. She felt tired all the time and often had difficulty sleeping. Eventually, the stress began to affect her resistance to illness. She caught colds and flu, which drained her resources even more. She was noticeably beginning to lose weight and her schoolwork was being affected.

It was at this time that the first symptoms of anorexia appeared. Amidst the chaos in the home, over which she had no control, she began to displace the focus of her attention to something over which she could have some control—her own person. She began to think that she was too fat and needed to be thinner. As time went on, these thoughts became increasingly obsessive and developed into an organized campaign. She started a program of exercises, fanatically counted calories, and began to put water on her cereal instead of high-calorie milk. She began to throw away the lunches that she brought to school, and lied about this to her mother. She began to "sleep through" meals and make rationalizations: "I'm too sick to eat tonight," or "I don't like what you're having for dinner." Although she denied her need for food, her body tried to protest to her mind, and resulted in constant thoughts about food and looking at pictures of food in magazines—as any starving person would. But she held fast to her control. She drank coffee because, "it filled me up without any calories." When her stomach began to be affected by the neglect, she switched to bland baby food or oatmeal with water when she did allow herself a controlled amount of food to eat.

Because of the weight loss and constant illness, June's mother took her to the family pediatrician. Suspicious, the doctor suggested that Mrs. S. keep a secret chart of what June was eating and report back after a week or two. When June discovered that her mother was keeping this check on her, she was furious at the intrusion into her affairs. Although it was unlike June to allow herself to overtly express anger, to her this was a critical situation. Both her adolescent independence and an important adjustment mechanism were being interfered with.

Much later, with the insights gained through therapy, June was able to understand what was going on psychologically during those months. Because of the turmoil created by the older brother she, the second eldest, assumed the role of the "good person," the compensator, so as not to add to the family problems. She thought that being emotionally responsible would somehow help the family regain control of a difficult situation. Her symptoms were a taking-on of the general family situation, and the result of turning her frustration and anger inward to keep it under control. This is a "good girl's" way. Her sickness also may have been a manifestation of her inner child, feeling deprived and frustrated, crying out for some of the attention that her older brother was monopolizing. The behavior may have been saying, "Hey!, don't forget about me; I'm a person too, and I need sympathy and attention also." Almost certainly an additional variable was her developing sexuality. She may have had reasons, which were never fully explored in our conversations, for wanting to deny the manifestations of her approaching womanhood.

At the time, however, no one understood what was going on. The family doctor, recognizing the evidence of psychological problems, referred June to a woman psychologist for counseling. Although this was an insightful referral to make, it may have come too late in the process, because the numerous weekly sessions seemed to produce no changes. June continued to become more depressed and less able or willing to respond to therapy. By the end of November she had lost 20 pounds and weighed only 85. She was becoming more introverted and emotionally isolated from everyone. By January, she had lost more weight, her menstrual periods had stopped, and she was beginning to lose her hair.

At this point, the psychologist referred June to another psychologist who was a specialist in eating disorders. The two-hour evaluation session with this psychologist was a difficult one for June. By this time, her body was no longer producing enough energy even to keep her warm, or to be able to think clearly. His questions probed areas of her personal life and history that she had been working hard to keep out of her consciousness. The complete shutdown of all of her emotions now generalized to her physical feelings, resulting in a general numbness. Even summoning the energy to speak was a labor. The consequence of this interview was a recommendation that June be hospitalized.

She was scheduled for an admission interview two weeks later, at a specialized anorexia section of a large hospital in the city. Those two weeks were difficult for June, and a time of mixed feelings. She knew that in the hospital, doctors would be working hard to interfere with and change her carefully controlled life-style—the only way she knew to cope with the difficult situations in her life—and this realization produced some reluctance and anxiety. On the other hand, she found herself feeling a sense of relief. The hospital would take off her shoulders the burden of responsibility she was too exhausted to carry any longer. She would be getting out of the home and could forget about it.

> At the time I did not care if I went to the hospital or did not go. I really did not care about anything at all. I felt isolated from everything around me—in a glass bubble. I could see the people on the outside but could not touch them. They were looking for something—digging—but could not find it. They could not hear me and I could not hear them.

She tried to eat during this time, but every attempt was defeated by the powerful compulsion. It would not release its hold; it was beyond her voluntary control. On the day that she was driven into the city for the admission evaluation interview at the hospital, accompanied by both her parents, her body weight was down to only 75 pounds.

> I found myself in a small empty conference room in Memorial Hospital. Sitting in front of me was a psychiatrist. My parents were on both sides of me for support. I did not need them. At least I thought I did not. They weren't there and neither was I. I did not take off my coat because it provided me with security and warmth. My hands were blue. I just sat staring at nothing, feeling completely numb. I could hear the voice of the doctor asking questions. "Why are you here? Why are you crying?" I was unaware of my tears. I could not answer. It was not that I did not want to answer—I could not physically speak. No words would come out.

By this time June was almost totally shut down, physically and emotionally. But what was the cause? And what was the effect? Was the emotional numbness a physiological consequence of her starvation? Or did the defense system, which was designed to blunt the intensity of her emotions, generalize to shut down the brain's ability to run the vital physical functions? Each comes from the same brain. June perceived her state this way:

> As my body shut down physically, my emotions turned off too. At this point I had lost all ability to feel anger, fear, or unhappiness. I deprived myself of feeling happy, healthy, proud, or good about myself. It was safer not to feel. I could not get close to or love anyone. I could not deal with or control these emotions, so I blocked them out. I beat the system.

It took only a few minutes for the doctor to make his decision. "We are going to admit her immediately," he said. Thus began a bizarre five-month game, in which the contestants were the patient and the health care system. At the end of the game we are left with an interesting rhetorical question: Was the patient the winner or the loser? June's time in the hospital was one of continuous conflict in both meanings of the word—internal and external. One side of her wanted to be a "good girl" and cooperate, but the other side was still dominant. She was the rebellious adolescent at its best—or worst. She rebelled against being deprived of her identity, against being just another case. She lied to the nurses and therapists, she manipulated everyone, and she cut school. She was beating the system by reasserting control of her life. She displayed much angry behavior during the initial period, and her prognosis was poor. When the hospital staff finally decided, as a last resort, to feed her through a tube to the stomach, she kicked, fought, and resisted in every way she could. But the maneuver accomplished its purpose. She agreed to eat rather than go through that ordeal again. However, when they set weekly weight-gain quotas, she carefully manipulated her food intake in order to just barely meet the objective. She was still managing to feel as if she was in control. As she realized later, she also was prolonging the time before she would have to go home again. Gradually, through a combination of continuous behavior modification, peer group therapy, and family therapy, June was ready to be released from the hospital in the middle of the summer. She was *physically* well again, but much hard work was still ahead.

Two of the developmental tasks of adolescence that had been put on hold now had to be dealt with in earnest and with a new honesty. The first was to learn how to deal with emotions in an open and mature manner. The second was to develop a more objective and healthy redefinition of her self-concept. She had to learn to accept that painful emotions are part of life and can be handled and experienced safely. She had already learned that the cost of denying emotions can be immense. Now, she had to accept that perfect is impossible, and that it is an unrealistic standard against which to evaluate self-worth.

> The first year that I was home I gradually let myself experience good feelings. This allowed me to feel better about myself and have some happy times. By the beginning of the second year at home I felt comfortable with family and friends. I started to let myself feel good without feeling guilty. I opened up more to others and became less shy.

June eventually began to date without fearing breakup and loss. She learned that these experiences did not have to be interpreted as potentials for personal rejection. She also learned that she did not have to please everyone. Being a pleaser is not a valid measure of self-worth. The ability to form close relationships evolved slowly but steadily as she learned that giving herself to another person did not mean that something was taken away. "I had been afraid to lose what little I had. Now I am not so afraid to love someone."

Allowing herself to experience negative emotions developed much later because it took longer to change the firmly set attitude that "good girls do not have bad feelings." In her senior year of high school, (what I call) that "unpredictable magic moment" seemed to arrive. The negative emotions were freed from their inhibitions relatively suddenly. As June described it, "The hurricane began to hit. I let myself become angry, really angry at others. For a while I honestly hated everyone." Although it was unpleasant, it was a relief and a valuable catharsis for her, and a healthy step forward. It represented a lesson that every one of us has to learn: not to hold anger inside for too long. Eventually this volcano will blow.

By the time June was finishing her second year of college, she had made healthy progress toward dealing more effectively with important life events and issues: fear, anxiety, the pressures of responsibilities, unhappiness, and loneliness. She learned to relax (somewhat) her striving for perfection in all things, and to feel better about herself as a person. "I am learning that I am not to blame for everything that happens around me. If the world comes to an end, it's not my fault."

She had become an attractive, pleasant person who was able to be a good friend. Only occasionally did I have to remind her to ease up and relax her intensity. As an indication of her psychological progress, and the fact that anorexia is behind her, we have this recent expression of her personal philosophy:

> Life is a pie. At one time the whole pie was food. Gradually other things—like roles, responsibilities, relationships, and life goals—assumed their normal sized sections of the pie. But food finally came to take its appropriate sized portion—only a little piece.

QUESTIONS FOR DISCUSSION

1. How do you feel about the social pressures that dictate what body shapes are attractive, or unattractive?
2. Do these pressures affect your behavior? In what way(s)?
3. How do they affect your self-image?
4. Do you think anorexia might be preventable? How?
5. Why do you suppose that anorexia is primarily a problem among American girls in the middle and upper social classes? What might be the causative factors that are unique to this culture?
6. I mentioned two adolescent developmental tasks on which June would belatedly have to resume work. Can you think of any others?

Chapter
10

Eating Disorder: Bulimia

What Goes Down Must Come Up

AMY O.: PURGE THE CONTAMINATION

Introduction

Do you know anyone, especially a young woman, whose eating behavior is a little strange or questionable? Have you discovered that she has a secret cache of junk food when she professes to be on a diet? Does she have an unusual lack of control when faced with a buffet display of food, or a chocolate cake, or a box of doughnuts? Have you noticed that she sometimes spends an unexplained length of time in the bathroom right after eating? Does she sometimes have dizzy spells, or stomach problems, or dental problems, or odd marks on her knuckles? Read on, for she may need your help.

Originally I had planned to write only one chapter on eating disorder. However, increased exposure to the nature and magnitude of the problem convinced me that there is much more information concerning these behavior patterns about which young women in particular need to be informed and forewarned. Eating disorders actually are even more complicated and poorly understood than I implied in Chapter 9. Some professionals bunch them all together under hyphenated headings, emphasizing their similar features and treatments. Others differentiate these disorders into a number of distinguishable patterns and focus on the differences. To the technical purist at least four pathologies center on abnormal eating behavior. In addition to anorexia nervosa, there is bulimia nervosa—alternate starving and binging/purging; bulimarexia—binging on large amounts of food followed immediately by induced vomiting or defecation; and simple bulimia—eating large amounts of food and getting very fat. *Bulimia* is a Greek word meaning, literally, ox hunger or eating like an ox.

In common practice, most professionals make just two major distinctions: anorexia nervosa and bulimarexia. The popular label for the second disorder, among professionals, is simply bulimia. This term is the one we will use in the following discussion. It is used interchangeably with bulimarexia in professional journals—referring to the same patterns of behavior. The disordered behavior being referred to can hardly be exaggerated, for it is truly bizarre when compared with normal eating behavior, if there is such a thing these days.

THE SYNDROME

A Brief Description

Here is a brief description of a somewhat typical bulimic pattern: A young college woman shares the attitude of the majority of the women she knows that she has to be thin to be attractive, and it is essential to look attractive. Because she often feels too heavy and not as attractive as she might be, she frequently musters her self-discipline and goes on a diet—usually overdoing it by skipping meals entirely or being too strict with the amount of food that she allows herself. This resolve is reinforced by her peers in the dance group or athletic team who admire commitment to the "right" body shape or weight and the disciplines of the program. Eventually, however, there is the inevitable failure of resolve. At times of stress and anxiety, or of disappointment, or depression and self-pity, and with the added impetus of her nagging hunger, she weakens and goes on a binge. This may be an entire large pizza, a half-gallon of ice cream, a box of doughnuts, several bags of junk food, or any combination of these things.

Her binge comes to an end only when the available food is gone, or her stomach is so painfully full that she cannot stuff any more food into it. This stage is followed immediately by strong feelings of guilt, failure, and self-deprecation. She considers herself weak; she has lost control; she has done a bad thing. She feels an overwhelming need to "clean herself out." She may take a strong laxative to induce diarrhea and purging. But this takes some time and may allow for the digestion of some of the food, and she will get fat. A faster way to purge is to bring it right back up the way it went down. This can be accomplished by sticking a couple of fingers down her throat to trigger the gag reflex and induce vomiting. Afterward she feels a great sense of relief and tension reduction. Any evidence of the occurrence she cleans up and hides, and the episode is over. As time goes on she repeats the cycle, satisfying her conflicting needs, and an adjustive habit becomes well established. Over time the pattern becomes more neurotic, obsessively occupying her thoughts, and the behavior becomes compulsively irresistible. She starts carefully planning the episodes— sometimes once a month, sometimes several times a week. She becomes like a chemically dependent person, an addict. In fact, she may mix in an occasional drinking or drug binge to ease some of the physical and emotional pain. Note that all of this is a secret of course, and she becomes more isolated psychologically, because she would be even more disappointed in herself if friends knew.

The first time that this full syndrome was described to me I simply shook my head; all I could think of was "weird," "bizarre." But my mind was also quickly filled with questions and a desire for explanations. Bulimia is complicated, and clinical psychology and medicine do not yet have all the answers, only a number of theories designed to help us understand and be able to offer assistance.

A More Comprehensive Description

There are some similarities, but also differences, between anorexics and bulimics. In Chapter 9 it seemed reasonable to refer to anorexic females as girls because they often start the disordered eating behavior early in puberty or before, and because of their physical immaturity. However, when talking about bulimics, it is more appropriate to refer to them as young women because the typical bulimic is older than the anorexic—usually between the ages of 18 and 30. It has been estimated (although making estimates of these numbers is difficult because of the secrecy factor of the disorder) that 15 to 25 percent of all women in this age group do some binging and purging. It is not a small population that we are talking about; in fact, bulimia may be a serious national health problem. Also, unlike anorexia, about 10 percent of bulimics are male. Many young men are involved in strict "make weight" sporting activities such as wrestling, boxing, and weight lifting, and may be on strict diets for a period of time, but may eat and drink all they wish in the off-season. Keep in mind that young men are also subjected to modern social attitudes regarding a slim, well-toned, physical ideal.

While both of these eating disorders involve a morbid, neurotic, and irrational fear of being fat, the two patterns of personality and behavior have some significant differences. Some anorexics may have occasional bulimic episodes, when hunger, depression, or self-pity causes them to fail in their dieting resolve. But these seldom occur and do not last very long. To the anorexic, eating much of anything, let alone large amounts of food, is abhorrent. On the other hand, bulimics rarely change or regress to a prolonged starvation pattern. They may occasionally fast, but the fast is invariably ended with binging and purging. For them binge eating has an attractive and reinforcing quality. It is an important part of the syndrome, and sometimes they carefully plan the next episode. While anorexics typically resemble the image of an emaciated concentration camp victim, bulimics tend to maintain a normal range of body weight. The fasting-binging-purging pattern only complicates their problem of trying to control their body weight. The body gets confused by the irregular and undependable intake of nutrition, so it stores fat as a protection. The result is a fluctuation of water weight only and an accumulation of fat. Little of nutrition value is gained and the body is weakened by deprivation, which leads to a further deterioration of self-worth resulting from another failure to maintain control.

Another shared consequence of these eating disorders is amenorrhea—irregular or no menstrual periods. A popular psychoanalytic explanation of this phenomenon is that it is a hysterical response to the anorexic's fear of and desire to deny and prevent her oncoming sexual maturation. This theory is weakened by recent research, however, that indicates that menstrual irregularities are almost the norm for all women who maintain life-styles involving strenuous exercise and low body weight. This psychoanalytic explanation is also unlikely to apply to bulimics, since a typical element in their personality patterns is an overstriving to achieve the social ideals of femininity.

There are other significant differences in the personalities of bulimic women. Typically they are older, more mature, and more socially and sexually experienced. They generally have high achievement motivation and aspire to high standards of performance—academically, athletically, or professionally. In fact, often they are successful in achieving high levels of performance because of their intelligence and competence, although often they are pursuing idealized standards of perfection. They are frequently regarded as "good girls" by their parents, teachers, and coaches. The irony is that little of this striving and achievement stems from any strong internalized set of values and beliefs. Rather, their behavior is directed primarily by their perception of the expectations of others. They are striving to conform, to please, and to be accommodating. They tend to have little or no clearly defined sense of who they are or what they stand for. They are desperately trying to achieve control and "perfection," without the support of any underlying attitude of "I think I can."

Thus, bulimics almost invariably labor under the burden of various anxieties: fear of failure or falling short of expectations, fear of being out of control and imperfect, fear of rejection or criticism, fear of the embarrassment of their bizarre eating patterns being discovered, and fear of never being able to change or extricate themselves from the hold of their obsessive-compulsive binging and purging. While this purging of the evidence of their uncontrolled gluttony is effective in reducing their anxiety and guilt, it is at the same time a reminder of their failure to maintain discipline and control. Disappointment, self-loathing, and depression are also common companions; and thoughts of suicide to end the hopeless cycle are not uncommon.

It is the custom in psychology to look for common factors in the background environments and histories of people with the same maladjustment pattern. With bulimia, there is far from universal agreement on what the common factors are or what their significance is. But the following are some of the common elements that seem to be significant as perceived by bulimics themselves.

The most significant factor seems to be the parent–child relationship. Women bulimics typically remember childhoods where one or both parents were dominating, demanding of high and strict standards of behavior and performance, and often overprotective. A high priority was placed on outward appearances and "the rules" for socially appropriate behavior. What a "good girl" is was not necessarily explained, but it was specifically defined: "A good girl eats everything on her plate and brushes her teeth after dinner." "A good girl does not talk back to adults." Even when there was agreement between the parents on priorities and values, they were conveyed to the daughter in different ways; the relationship with each parent was very different. The father often was perceived as a strong personality. He held great power to reinforce the girl's behavior and attitudes with praise and punishment, although he seldom directly used either one. He was perceived as distant and difficult to approach. In fact, he may not have been in the home very much. There was little, if any, emotional closeness between father and daughter. Pleasing her father was important to the bulimic, but she rarely received any feedback to tell her that she had done so.

On the other hand, pleasing the mother was easy. All the girl had to do was conform to perfectionist standards and obey the rules: Dress properly, speak properly, be on time for dinner, observe bedtime rituals, and bring home from school the right kind of report card. Bulimic women usually recall mixed feelings toward their mothers. They appreciated and respected that their mothers were conscientious homemakers. Mother was always there and always doing what should be done. When older, they may even have sympathized with what they suspected was the mother's frustration at not having the opportunity for a personal or professional career. But they also resented the overprotection, the domination, and the inflexible standards of performance.

The result of this childhood environment is sometimes a teenage girl who emerges into young womanhood with little sense of readiness or competence. She feels overdominated and controlled, even smothered. She senses strong pressure to perform and achieve at a high level, but little of the motivation comes from her own internal and personal needs—except to have the approval of others by being passively accommodating. She has little sense of a personal identity, and feels almost no control over her life.

The organized, almost ritualized, binging and purging that she falls into provides this sense of control over something in her life. It also provides a dependably adjustive, albeit very nonintegrative, control of her troublesome anxieties. As with all nonintegrative adjustments, the cost is usually tremendous. The short-range adjustment produces long-range maladjustment. To repeat, the bulimic's behavior and psychological condition are not unlike that of a chemically dependent person, and like the addict, the long-range consequences can be severe and/or life-threatening.

Effects of Bulimia on Physical Health

Bulimarexia can cause long-range physical effects, as well. Surely you remember the unpleasant, sharp, bilious taste in your mouth after you threw up from being sick. The liquid in the stomach consists of strong acids, secreted there to digest food. Repeated exposure of the tissues in the mouth to these acids can cause painful ulcers and blisters. The acids can also dissolve the enamel on the teeth, making them more susceptible to cavities and toothbrush wear. Inserting fingers in the mouth to trigger the vomit reflex can cause scratches in the roof of the mouth and abrasions on the knuckles, and those same stomach acids will make the throat sore and may cause the voice to become rough and raspy. The muscle spasms involved in vomiting also have been known to cause hernias. The whole gastrointestinal system can become so messed up that the bulimarexic will develop ulcers or even a ruptured stomach, which can be fatal. Frequent purging will cause serious disruption of the body's electrolyte balance—particularly potassium deficiency—resulting in anemia, lethargy, and weakness. It is particularly dangerous to deprive the heart of the chemical nutrients necessary for it to function efficiently. Electrolyte deficiencies can cause kidney failure and urinary tract infections. Also affected is the endocrine system and its production of the various hormones necessary for normal function. The most noticeable example is the disruption of menstrual cycles. Obviously, bulimic purging can have very serious long-range consequences.

The questions remain: What starts some people on such a bizarre, compulsive, and self-destructive pattern of behavior? How can they stop it? The clinical literature provides us with some clues. The initial binging episodes have some common themes. The most obvious is simply an immature, self-indulgent response to the hunger of a strict diet. The woman gives in to the inner child crying that it is hungry, and the child wins. Anxiety is a common trigger. It is easy to learn that eating eases the stomach discomfort that accompanies anxiety. It is not unusual for a young woman to respond to disappointment or rejection in a romantic relationship by overeating. Related causes are depression or boredom. There is a widely held theory that some metabolic systems react to certain foods in a manner not unlike the way that an alcoholic reacts to alcohol differently from other people. Once started they cannot stop. The most common of these foods contain white flour and/or white sugar. For example, doughnuts are on most compulsive eaters' bad list.

Curing this disabling compulsion requires much the same treatment as that for anorexia. It involves careful behavior modification, individual insight psychotherapy, and group and family therapy. At best, it is a long process with uneven progress. Frequent slips and regressions are common. By herself, a bulimic cannot do what is required; she requires help. Attitudes are difficult to change, and these young women have to modify a number of irrational attitudes. They have to change their feelings about food and eating. They have to develop a more realistic perception of their bodies' appearance. Most difficult of all, they need to build an entirely new concept of their personal identities, and of their competence and self-worth. They have to internalize a personal set of values, and become more autonomous and less dependent on the opinions and expectations of others.

The Case of Amy O.

Amy was certain that it was only a matter of time before she was discovered. The humiliation and embarrassment would be unbearable. She was aware of the group of six girls on the floor above her in the dorm who had made a fad of binge and purge parties. She had heard rumors that these were "humongous pig-outs," with competitions on who could eat the most in two hours. But Amy was also aware that other people who knew about the activities of this group delighted in ridiculing them behind their backs. They were the laughing stock of the dorm. And somehow she just did not fully trust the only other person who knew about her own eating habits—her roommate, Wendy. It was Wendy, in fact, who had taught her about the guilt-reducing effects of a quick, self-induced throwing up—to "clean out the bad stuff" and keep from getting fat. It was Wendy's general lack of morals and ethics that was the basis of Amy's mistrust. How could someone with such a complete lack of respect for other people's rights be trusted to keep a confidence? Amy often wondered to herself how two people with the same illness could be such different personalities. Wendy had no inhibition whatever about shoplifting food or other personal items. She would even steal money to buy food if the opportunity presented itself. Amy's own thoroughly instilled ideas of what a good person is never allowed her even to consider such behavior. She could remember several occasions when Wendy had coveted a box of doughnuts or cookies that was too large to hide in her clothing. She would check to see that no one was looking and then simply open the box, stuff the goodies into her mouth as fast as she could chew and swallow, and then hide the near-empty box back on the shelf. Amy would always move to another part of the store so as not to be associated with Wendy.

It wasn't that Wendy was a bad person. In fact, Amy and she were close friends and had shared many confidences. Amy excused Wendy's "me-first" selfishness as understandable given her rough childhood. While Wendy's father spoiled her by giving her everything she wanted, he was never able to give her any love, except the wrong kind. From the time she was about nine years old, he had used and abused her sexually. It always occurred when he was drunk and when her mother was out working as a night nurse, which she did about once a week. These awful experiences finally ended when Wendy was 14. Her mother had discovered some suspicious indications and gently but thoroughly questioned the girl. The father was summarily thrown out of the home by a court order, and the parents were divorced a few months later. Wendy had rarely seen or heard from her father in the following years. Amy wondered if Wendy would ever be able to resolve her conflicted and confused feelings about sex, about relationships with men, and particularly about the concept of "pleasing" men.

Such musings and wonderings were not isolated occurrences for Amy. It seemed that her head was constantly full of questions, and she frequently found that she was silently talking to herself. She was grateful that her own childhood had not been the horror show that Wendy's had been. But it hadn't been any bouquet of roses either, at least not as she had perceived and experienced it. It couldn't have been, she thought, or both she and Wendy wouldn't have the same neurotic obsession with food and fatness, and the same bizarre compulsion to binge and purge food, in spite of the obvious costs and consequences to their bodies and minds. "Why do we do this to ourselves? Why can't we stop? How did it all begin?" she asked herself.

It was difficult for Amy to remember when the whole pattern of eating, fatness and thinness, weighing herself, disgust with the image in the mirror, and overconcern with other people's opinions was not a tension-filled preoccupation. "Ten! Something changed when I was ten," she recalled. Before that all the signals said, "Isn't she tiny and cute." That was good. That was acceptable. That was the basis for a comfortable relationship with her two older brothers, grandmother, aunts, and uncles, and with Dad. But during the summer of the year that she turned 10, between the fourth and fifth grades, something changed. "Instead of going to a cabin in the mountains, we went on a vacation trip and ate out a lot; I gained ten pounds and grew a few inches. I began to mature, and my nipples were swollen. I wasn't tiny and cute anymore; I was ugly."

It had been OK to be a tomboy when she was tiny and cute. But now her older brothers seemed to think her competitive efforts were funny, and they began to tease her. She was unsure how to act. She began to be apprehensive about her father's sarcastic insults—like those he directed at her mother when she put on a few pounds. "Lard ass" and "saddlebags" were typical comments. As Amy said several times, "He could be a sarcastic son of a bitch when he wanted to, especially when he was drinking." Even though some of the weight gain was muscle, which she could use to her advantage, she saw it as chubby and ugly. How could one be active and muscular and have fun without being unattractive? The social dictum—be lean and thin, fat is ugly—also suggested the solution. She began to eat lightly at meals. Eating less must be the answer. This wasn't easy when her mother insisted, "You must start the day with a good breakfast," and "Finish all of your dinner." But at school she wasn't so closely supervised, and she could throw away half or even all of her lunch. Thus, Amy's eating disorder had its genesis as far back as the fifth or sixth grade. As her body began its change from cute little girl into that of a young woman, these unwelcome changes were out of her control. Limiting her food intake was a small measure, but it was one thing she could control.

Looking back, Amy realized how important a role her father played in all of this turmoil. To the young adolescent woman, her father's approval, acceptance, and attention seemed to be very important. But little of any of these was given. His job kept him on the road about half of the time, and when he was home, his routine was to settle down with a drink or two, have supper, have a couple more drinks, and be asleep half-way through the evening. Furthermore, he had no capacity for emotional closeness and wanted little involvement in the details of family life. For Amy's needs, her father was unavailable.

Amy's older brothers had much less difficulty getting Dad's attention. Their athletic prowess through high school and his natural interest in athletics gave them plenty to talk about. They also spent many hours together as they helped him put an addition onto the back of the house and periodically tinkered with the car. But Amy wasn't included in any of these activities; she was only a girl.

In junior high school Amy became involved in gymnastics and track. This interest was probably motivated initially by the need to identify with, and be included in, the areas that got attention and approval by the males in the family. However, she continued to be a highly dedicated participant in gymnastics and track through high school and college—for reasons that were more subtle and personal and more difficult to understand and explain. Serious gymnastics and middle-distance running demand great self-discipline and dedication of time. Life is very structured. The body becomes a highly tuned and toned machine, requiring constant attention. Body weight is checked on the scales several times a day. Both sports have high standards of perfection. World-class gymnasts and runners receive much media attention and public adulation. The bodies of most of these women are beautifully toned and lean. But they are also small and have little or nothing of the normal female roundedness on the chest and hips. Thus, these sports provided ideal outlets for Amy's needs. She threw herself into the organized activities of gymnastics and track, depending on the season, with total dedication. Even weekends and off-season she ran or rode her bike every day, doing sit-ups, exercising, checking her weight, and setting incremental weight-loss goals of several ounces a day. These activities provided the perfect rationalization for her hidden neurotic goals. After all, "The good athlete trains all of the time, the ideal athlete is thin and muscular; there is no fat." Amy even went to gymnastics camp during the summers between high school sessions so that she could stay in the supervised and disciplined environment of organized athletics.

But these idealized goals of physique and weight are difficult to achieve and maintain. The body's natural mechanisms of homeostasis fight back. It is normal for an adolescent girl to develop hips, breasts, and begin her menstrual periods. (Amy still had not experienced her first menstrual period by her senior year of high school.) The enormous growth and development processes of adolescence require plenty of good nutrition and create the infamous hunger of the adolescent. So fighting these powerful natural processes is, in the long run, a losing proposition. Trying to achieve her unnatural standards of perfection for leanness was bound to result in a sense of failure. A person more directed by external influences than by internalized values is eventually going to buckle under the pressure of the frequent or chronic sense of failure, and just give up.

Amy's bulimarexic behavior actually began in just such a circumstance at gymnastics camp during the summer before she turned 16. At camp the physical discipline and regimen were somewhat more relaxed than "in season." A highlight for any camper was the arrival of the "goody box" from home. Amy's mother, also a perfectionist, was a first-class baker of cookies.

The day that a box of her special chocolate-chip cookies arrived at camp coincided with one of Amy's low-morale/ready-to-quit moods. (Ironically, breakdown of resolve can be just as extreme and unreasoning as overstrict self-discipline.) To her own amazement Amy mindlessly and compulsively ate the entire box at a sitting. No sharing, no saving some for later. Also to her surprise, the psychological reaction was dreadful. She stared at the empty box and was immediately overwhelmed with a sense of guilt and failure. Worse than just overeating, cookies are a "bad food," dirty, equated with fat. Desperate to undo the mistake and regain control, and to prevent all of those cookies from being turned into fat, she took several doses of laxative. She subsequently had to make several unpleasant trips to the camp toilet throughout that night.

Coincidentally, this also was the summer that Amy met and established a friendship with Wendy. When Amy privately shared her miseries with Wendy the next day, she was surprised at the matter-of-fact nature of the friend's response: "Oh, you don't need to go to all that trouble, silly, just stick your finger down your throat and throw it all up. It's much faster and easier, and nothing has time to get digested." As disgusted as she was at the thought, the idea stayed in the back of her mind. The next time she "slipped," and ate a box of candy bars, she quietly went off into the woods and made herself throw up the evidence of her transgression. As she cleaned herself and rinsed the bilious taste from her mouth and throat, Amy was amazed at how calm and peaceful she felt. Gone along with the stomach sickness from the sugar overdose were the anxiety, guilt, and self-condemnation. Everything was made right. "Everything is OK now," she thought, "and it won't happen again."

But it did happen again, of course—several times. With each repetition the tension-reducing quality of purging became further reinforced in her mind. The tranquil, adjusted state became a goal in its own right, and the binging-purging pattern became the adjustment mechanism to achieve it. Amy did not understand what was going on and she felt strange and frightened. She felt caught in the paradox of having less and less control over a behavior pattern that had the concomitant function of controlling her anxieties. She also was confused about how and why she was different from Wendy, who was doing the same thing. Wendy's behavior seemed less complicated. For her, purging was simply a device to keep her weight under control. But for Amy, vomiting came to have a purpose of its own. The cycle seemed to be triggered by a buildup of tension, not hunger. Once the habit was established she began to plan ahead for the next episode, not unlike the addict planning for the next drink or fix. The first successful scheme was at camp that summer. Instead of going to the next group activity, she sometimes volunteered for after-meal cleanup. This way she could surreptitiously stuff herself with leftovers and then go to the deserted toilet house to purge.

Like all neurotic compulsive adjustments, this one was maintained at considerable personal cost. As the habit continued through the years, Amy came to hate it desperately. She hated its control over her, and she hated feeling weird and not able to understand what was going on. While each purge session was tension relieving, the gluttonous binging part of the pattern was another failure to be able to control her eating. She hated that feeling of failure and being disappointed in herself yet another time. Contrary to what we would expect, Amy's bulimia did not interfere with her athletic success. Her compulsive motivation to achieve at a superior level was powerful enough to keep her from binging/purging during the competitive season, even though she found herself thinking about it quite often. She had to be able to perform well and could not endanger her health and strength reserves. In addition, the strenuous activity burned up so many calories that her weight was kept low and she worried less about fatness. And exercise also reduced tension.

But there were many weeks at a time during the school years that Amy seemed under the total control of the binge-purge obsession. Almost no decisions, in the course of a day, were made without the influence of this dominating need. She had to organize and plan each day to provide opportunities for private throwing up. She kept careful mental records of the times during the day when bathrooms were most likely to be empty. Whenever she was away from her room or her home, she always made sure that she knew where the nearest bathroom was. This was important because she would literally become panicky if too much time were passing since she had eaten. Too much food was being allowed to digest. Her preferred places to vomit provided either assured isolation and secrecy or else good cover noise—such as a running bathtub or shower. On junk-food buying sprees, she was careful never to shop in just one place, so that no one could see how much she was buying. In this regard, being a college woman on a strict budget had its handicaps. One could easily blow $30 or $40 at a time on "nasty food," and she rarely had that kind of money. But $10 or $12 could go a long way with careful planning.

Binge food had to meet an even more important criterion than price. It literally had to be "bad" or "nasty," forbidden on a normal healthy or training diet. The important ingredients were high proportions of sugar, salt, flour, or fat. The neurotic satisfaction increased if the bad food also resulted in a particularly nasty, unpleasant vomit—in other words, if it was especially punishing. But being a college student also had some advantages—particularly if you were served by a cafeteria where you could eat all you wanted for one price. Both Amy and Wendy became skillful at returning for two, three, or four refills of their trays, while not letting anyone realize what they were doing. This involved sitting in different places each time and not returning to the same servers.

Several times during our conversations, Amy commented that the story of their college eating adventures would make a fascinating movie. But how would you label it in the movie guide—horror, thriller, mystery? Certainly not a comedy! Although some of the capers could be made funny in the telling, the visual scenes of binging and purging would be ugly and repulsive. Amy and Wendy specialized in hosting take-out parties in their room—knowing that the wasteful habits of some of their friends would provide ample leftovers. Cold, greasy leftover pizza, for example, made a particularly repulsive

binge and a really nasty vomit. On more than one occasion the two girls secretly recovered from the dorm dumpster the throwaways from other
people's take-outs, such as half-empty boxes of Chinese food. Although not as
convenient as pizza, this too could be eaten by the handful, right out of the
box. On two occasions Amy devised a scheme for a cheap, private binge
without having to go out and buy junk food. She would bake her own cake or a
big batch of cookies. But she eventually abandoned this plan as unsuccessful,
because on both occasions, before she could get the recipe to the bake pans,
she ate the entire bowl of raw, uncooked batter.

There were good times and bad times, strong times and weak times.
There would be totally "lost weekends" and then weeks without a binge-
purge episode. It seemed to depend on her moods, or the opportunity or
availability of food, or the amount of stress or tension that she was under. Amy
tried many times in many ways to bring the compulsion under control with
highly structured and disciplined diets and eating schedules. It wasn't as
straightforward as the solution to an alcoholic's problem—to completely ab-
stain from alcohol. After all, one has to eat. Amy could never get the urge to
throw up entirely out of her mind. She would try to be strong, to hold out.
But tension would gradually build and build, and she would eventually give
up. It was demoralizing to feel so little in control over what was going on in
her life. Her tricks and devices, like secretly carrying a toothbrush at all times
to try to protect her teeth, seemed pathetically inadequate compared to the
scope of the problem.

When burdened with a seemingly interminable problem, everyone will
try to maintain hope, and to fend off the depression of hopelessness, by trying
to visualize the end of the travail. We have all found ourselves saying: "It will
be all over when. . . . " It is much easier to marshal psychological resources for
a finite length of time. The thought of having to endure a particular stress
forever is intolerable. Amy decided that the key elements in her compulsive
illness were probably the strict disciplines of her athletic activities and the
heavy academic demands and stresses of college. "I will be all better when I
am finished with college."

But at the end of her senior year, when the year's competitions and exams
were over for the last time, there was that awful two- or three-week period
before graduation with nothing to do but think about the future. The highly
structured situation was no longer there to direct her each day. There were
dreadful attacks of anxiety as Amy realized that there were no more road
signs. "Where do I go now?" There were no more specific social instructions
except: "You are on your own now; go out into the world and be successful."
Amy wanted to cry out: "But what do I do? I don't know how to decide these
things. I don't even know who I am." Perhaps most frightening was the
realization that the old obsessions were not fading away. In fact, triggered by
the new insecurities, the old compulsions emerged as strong as ever, as adjustive habits are conditioned to do.

During this period of time came, in a way, the magic moment of truth; her
dysfunction was no longer avoidable. She was forced to face the fact that the

bulimic pattern of behavior was a symptom of her problems rather than a solution. Further, she was forced to admit that it was beyond her ability to control it by herself. She could not bear the thought of living the rest of her life in this manner, but she would need help to change it. Amy decided to share her problem with one of her coaches, with whom she had become close over the four years. Her coach was not unfamiliar with bulimia after coaching women athletes for many years, and listened to Amy's story with sympathy and understanding. Because Amy was still eligible for college support services, the coach immediately made an appointment for her with the director of the college counseling services. The psychologist was able to spend several hours talking with Amy that week. They decided together that Amy should be admitted as an outpatient to the eating disorders clinic in a nearby city. She was able to start in a program of therapy almost immediately. And thus began the most difficult but important year of her life. She did not go home that summer; instead, she found a full-time job to enable her to attend her therapy sessions two or three times a week. Therapy consisted of individual psychotherapy and group sessions with other bulimics. Amy was too far from home for family therapy, and she was certain that her father would never have considered getting involved.

The year was a difficult one for several reasons, for Amy was combining insight psychotherapy with her first year of being on her own—a pretty tough assignment. In Amy's case she had to let go of and change a compulsive neurotic life-style and, at the same time, catch up with the long postponed adolescent task of deciding who she was and what she wanted to be. Fortunately, she had some strong assets working in her favor. The intelligence, stamina, perseverance, and drive for success that she honed during her years of academic and athletic labor combined to keep her going during the times when she wanted to quit. Toward the end of a year of therapy and living on her own, she found that she could look at her present self in the mirror, and at what she wanted for herself in the future, with much more clarity, objectivity, and optimism than had ever been possible before. The bulimic compulsion was no longer a serious problem, because it was no longer needed. She was no longer obsessed with fatness or with what other people were thinking about her. The few extra pounds that came with maturing and the cessation of a strenuous athletic program did not bother her. Amy even surprised herself with the new independence of her thinking: "Who cares what they think! It's my body and I have to live with it. Anyone who is really my friend will not be looking for things to criticize."

It was also becoming clear to Amy that she wanted a professional career, and that it would require a graduate degree. After that, she could see herself ready for marriage and a family. She realized that she was not yet completely well and there was much more work to do. She was cautiously aware, in fact, that she might always have to be careful when confronted by a buffet of "bad" foods. When I last saw Amy, then about three years out of college, she said, "I'm OK now—finally!"

When I asked Amy what she had heard lately from Wendy, her expression changed. This, unfortunately, was a different story. Wendy clearly remained trapped in the cycle of compulsive bulimia, but was still unwilling to admit that she had a problem. Whenever Amy tried to bring up the subject, out of concern for her friend, Wendy responded with annoyance and resentment. The two women had little to talk about anymore, and communicated less and less as time went on. Amy was aware, however, that Wendy had been hospitalized several times for serious gastrointestinal problems, including an ulcer, and a troublesome kidney disorder, and for injuries incurred in an automobile accident after she fainted while driving her car. Amy was saddened at the deterioration of her friend, but felt helpless, for Wendy would accept no help. She often thought quietly to herself: "There but for the grace of God. . . . "

QUESTIONS FOR DISCUSSION

1. What details surprised you as you read and learned about this eating disorder?
2. Whether you grew up in the same cultural environment and experienced similar social pressures or not, can you identify with or understand some of the background factors which contribute to this maladjustment?
3. You probably know a bulimic person, even if you're not aware of it. Do you think you will be able to recognize the signs or symptoms after reading this chapter?
4. If you had reason to suspect that a friend of yours was bulimic, what would you do? What would you not do?
5. If you learned that Amy was coming to your school to give a talk with a question session afterward, what would you like to ask her?

Chapter
11

Gender-Identity Adjustment: Homosexuality

The So-called Insult to Nature

ROBERTO V.: WHY AM I DIFFERENT?

Introduction

What are your feelings as you begin this assigned reading? Are you looking forward to it? Or do you begin with a reluctant and resentful attitude, resulting in attempts to think of an excuse to do something else? These questions are necessary in order to clear the air of personal bias. It is the obligation of good social scientists (and good social science students) to pursue the answers to questions about behavior with objectivity and open-mindedness. Many Americans find it difficult to discuss the subject of homosexuality without bias and with subjective feelings and/or ignorance. It has been my experience that on the day when my class has been asked to read a case study and come prepared to discuss the subject of homosexuality, as many as half of them will be missing from class. Those remaining usually have an interesting and useful class discussion. In case you are feeling some reluctance, let us begin with a quiz.

Answer true or false to each of the following statements:

1. Homosexuals represent only a very small proportion of our population.
2. In terms of sexual preference, a person is either heterosexual or homosexual. You have to be one or the other.
3. Homosexuals are easily recognized because gay men are always effem-

inate and "swishy" and lesbian women are always masculine and "butchy."

4. It is justifiable to be suspicious of a man's sexuality if he is a hair-dresser, a musician, an artist, or in the theater, or if a woman is an outstanding athlete, has well-defined muscles, likes to wear pants, or wears her hair very short.

5. Homosexuality is a mental illness. Psychologists have confirmed that homosexuals are invariably maladjusted and unhappy.

6. Homosexuals usually have hostile feelings toward the opposite sex and therefore should be considered dangerous, especially around children.

7. Homosexuals are likely to try to convert other people to their sexual orientation, so it is safer to avoid them and, to repeat, keep them away from children.

You can calculate your score on this quiz simply by counting the number of statements to which you responded false. These are all incorrect statements, even though they are all beliefs that are widely held by people in the United States.

Why is there such widespread misunderstanding about homosexuality and such strong social feelings on the subject? People naturally have a curiosity about a need that is as strong and persistent as sex. One's sexuality is also an important part of the self-concept. So people need to know what is normal and "OK." Unfortunately, for most of history, science has done little to provide accurate and valid answers to these questions. Thorough and scientifically objective study of human sexuality is only about 40 years old. While the ground-breaking research of Kinsey, Masters and Johnson, and others has done much to clear away our ignorance, many questions remain. Thus, it is reasonable to ask, If sexual interaction between males and females (heterosexuality) is the more usual or "natural" form, because of its procreative function, then why are some people sexually attracted to others of the same sex (homosexuality)? Science does not yet know the answer(s) to this question, although there are several prevailing theories.

But before we can discuss the statements on the quiz, we have to clarify some of the terms that are in common use by scientific authorities. Even here, arriving at definitions that are universally acceptable is difficult. Categorizing the sexual orientation of people is not as simple or clear-cut as people tend to think it is.

Definitions

To start, *what* is a homosexual? Or *who* is a homosexual? Masters, Johnson, and Kolodny define a homosexual as "a person who has a preferred sexual attraction to people of the same sex over a significant period of time." In this form it is a noun. The word is also an adjective when it describes the *behavior* of engaging in overt sexual relations with another person of the same sex. But how do we label a person who is attracted to the same sex, but who never acts on this attraction? Or a person who is basically heterosexual in orientation but has same-sex relations when no opposite-sex partner is available (such as in prison)? There are also people who can be aroused by either sex or who have sexual relations with both sexes. These people, *bisexuals*, comprise at least a third category of human sexual orientation. Thus, homosexual can be a state of mind or an attitude, or a pattern of behavior.

Incidence

The best available statistics on the distribution of different patterns of sexual preference and behavior in the United States are still the studies done by Kinsey et al. in the 1940s. The most surprising revelation of these studies was that exclusive heterosexuality and exclusive homosexuality are only the opposite ends of a continuum. In between these extremes Kinsey placed five patterns of bisexuality that were different according to the relative amount of preference for one sex or the other. The number of people who indicated that they were exclusively homosexual was approximately 5–10 percent of males and 3–5 percent of females. This number appears to be consistent throughout all Western cultures regardless of socioeconomic, ethnic, racial, or geographical variables. The total number of bisexuals is at least equal to the number of homosexuals. Based on these numbers, how many people in the United States would identify themselves as something other than heterosexual? Tens of millions of people have made distinct choices of sexual orientation and preference that are not only contrary to cultural norms but also have been actively discouraged and punished, for all of our history, by the law, religious doctrine, and the fear and hostility of society as a whole. Certainly, homosexuality is not a rare phenomenon, and human sexuality in general is obviously not a clear either/or matter.

As far as we can tell, homosexuality has always been part of human behavior; and at this time it is apparently a part of every known society, in spite of widely differing degrees of acceptance or rejection. In the United States, and probably in most developed countries, the homosexual subculture is a large, well-organized social system, with all of the components of the larger heterosexual society—including newspapers and other publications, religious organizations, counseling services, vacation resorts, and medical facilities. All this information puts considerable strain on long-held popular attempts to judge what is "normal" or "abnormal" regarding human sexuality—except from a purely statistical point of view.

The increasing openness and visibility, over the last two decades, of the large homosexual subculture within our society should have made it obvious by now that quiz questions 3 and 4 are inaccurate stereotypes. These stereotypes have been perpetuated by moviemakers, entertainers, and popular superstition. As we become more aware of the number of homosexuals who are movie stars, military heros, professional athletes, holders of public office, and members of all occupations—oftentimes they are people whom "we never would have suspected"—we realize that there is no typical homosexual occupation, homosexual behavior or appearance, or homosexual life-style. The homosexual "world" is every bit as complex and varied as the heterosexual world.

What are the real differences then, and why do they cause so much anxiety and hostility in so many people? We must return to our definition question of what a homosexual is. Scientific study of this question in recent history has been virtually dominated by medicine, psychiatry, and psychology. From their early years, these sciences regarded it as an illness, an abnormality, and a problem. From this starting point, research was naturally directed toward discovering what was the cause and how to "cure" the problem. At the start of this century homosexuality was assumed to be an abnormality or illness with which a person was born. In the ensuing decades psychiatry and psychology turned to a theory that it was a developmental problem resulting from an adverse parent–child relationship and could therefore be cured by appropriate therapy. A very low cure rate eventually caused this theory to be questioned and stimulated research into many other aspects of the heredity vs. environment conundrum. These new directions of research have included theories of inappropriate hormone influence, social conditioning, and genetic abnormalities. Unfortunately, all of the research to date remains inconclusive. We still do not know what causes one to become a homosexual— or, for that matter, a heterosexual. But research goes on and theoretical debates continue with great enthusiasm. I encourage you to do additional reading of your own into the details of recent research into prenatal hormone influences on the development of male brains and female brains, and into family relationships. There is a short bibliography at the end of this chapter.

To their credit, the sciences of psychiatry and psychology have officially changed earlier beliefs about homosexuality when objective research proved them to be false. Homosexuality as a category of clinical or mental illness was discarded by the APA in 1974; with the publishing of *DSM IIIR* it was no longer listed as such. This decision was preceded by a number of impressive psychological studies that showed that homosexuality is not inherently a psychological illness, that as a behavior its forms are as varied as heterosexual behavior, and that the majority of homosexuals are well adjusted and productive with no sign of psychiatric illness. In fact, the incidence of mental illness or maladjustment among homosexuals is no higher than that among heterosexuals.

Such data were no doubt received by psychology professionals with amazement, considering the immense weight of social pressures that work against a homosexual person being able to form a comfortable sense of self-worth or to win the struggle against feelings of inferiority. For centuries society's pervasive homophobia has manifested itself in the form of ridiculing jokes, derogatory names, stigmatizing, job discrimination, persecution, punishment by the law, ostracism from religious organizations, and every other imaginable form of hostility and anxious defensiveness.

Of course, some homosexuals do become maladjusted. Stop and think for a minute how you would handle such powerful negative social attitudes against your sexual preference. At the least, it is always difficult for a young homosexual to deal with such decisions as "coming out," the desire to couple, the formation of a personal family, and the coming to terms with one's mortality—of which the modern (AIDS) crisis provides a constant reminder. But some of their mental illnesses can be serious, with the not uncommon consequences of psychotic thinking, depression, suicidal tendencies, or substance abuse and addiction. Additionally, psychiatry distinguishes two particular maladjustments that can involve problems with sexual orientation:

Gender-identity disorder, in which the person's physical sex is different from his or her gender identity (sense of being male or female), and in which the person has difficulty adjusting to this contradiction.

Transsexualism, a more serious gender-identity disorder in which a person feels trapped in the body of the wrong sex. Transsexualism can create a very difficult adjustment problem and often results in the desire to have one's physical gender altered by surgery.

While we are discussing maladjustments associated with homosexuality, it is necessary to acknowledge another group of people who receive much less attention and assistance than homosexuals. These are the families of homosexuals. Mothers, fathers, brothers and sisters, and others are often confronted with great turmoil of thoughts and feelings upon learning that they have a homosexual in the family. They often feel shame and embarrassment and are anxious about what other people will think. It is typical to want to keep this information from public knowledge. An unfortunate by-product of the long-held psychiatric theory that homosexuality primarily had its origins in poor parent–child relationships is that parents feel shame, guilt, and remorse—with prolonged lamenting about "What did I do wrong?"

Fortunately, the opportunities for positive assistance with these adjustment problems are more readily available than in former years. Not only are most counselors and therapists less encumbered by outdated theoretical models than in earlier decades, but there are now several types of well-organized support groups available for those families willing to reach out for assistance. One of the best of these is PFLAG, Parents and Friends of Lesbians and Gays, which is a national organization.

The Case of Roberto V.

Roberto's story is somewhat typical of those which have been told to me over the years on occasions when students were either comfortable enough with their lives to share them with me or so uncomfortable they needed to share their feelings and questions with someone they believed they could trust.

Sometime during the spring of the year that he was 13, Roberto awoke one morning from a particularly vivid dream with feelings he described as "a startling revelation." He had discovered (or accepted) a word to label the confused thoughts and feelings he had "been aware of for as long as he could remember." The word was *homosexual*. Although he had an incomplete understanding of what this word meant, he somehow knew it was the right word to describe what he had been feeling. In the dream Roberto was 16 and had selected the momentous occasion of his birthday to *announce* to his parents the truth of his secret preference. He apparently had chosen 16 as the appropriate age because his sister was 16 and she seemed mature by comparison.

During the next three years, his adolescence began to run its course in earnest. As sexuality became a larger part of his personality, his feelings intensified and sexual fantasies became more frequent. He found himself increasingly more attracted to males and less attracted to females. He became disturbed and confused because his reactions were "not what they were supposed to be." He had hoped that the revelation in the dream was only a dream or a passing phase. But with the passage of time it became more of a reality. However, his thoughts and feelings remained private and secret. He did not forget the dream and, in fact, awaited his sixteenth birthday with some anxious anticipation. This was to be the magic moment when he could finally be honest with his parents about his feelings and be free of the "burden." Burdens are so much heavier when carried alone! Since Roberto did not look different or act differently from other boys, there was little danger of being discovered and teased by his peers. Nevertheless, his fantasies included the fear that somehow someone would be able to read his mind and then ridicule and embarrass him.

Roberto's first sexual encounter was with a male classmate when he was 14. Although both teenagers considered the relationship to be casual, it lasted for two years. He described the sexual activity as "sex games and experimentation," which allowed him to believe that it was probably just a phase that they would soon pass through. The friend also "played these games" with several other boys. But, as Roberto assessed the situation, he was the only one who "did not escape unscathed." While the sex games seemed to satisfy the sexual fantasies of the other boys, "they wound up only teasing and enticing mine." This was not a satisfying situation at all for Roberto. For the next three years, he went into a period of abstinence from sex and denial of his homosexual desires. It was a period of loneliness but of less conflict. The "big 16" birthday arrived—and passed. He still did not have the courage to tell anyone, including his parents. Instead of "coming out," he became more secretive and introverted. His true desires remained private. The high school years were in general a difficult time for Roberto. He felt so different and "out of it"—unable to become involved in the coupling activities of his peers and their frequent conversations about sex. He often was tempted to join in their activities just to be "normal" and fit in. However, coupling with a boy was out of the question and the idea of going out with girls did not feel right.

When he was 19, he finally decided that the best way to break out of this homosexual "stage" was to attempt to establish relationships with women. This plan was facilitated by the availability of large numbers of young women at a nearby coed junior college where he was enrolled as a commuting day student. For a while these heterosexual activities proved to have some positive consequences. He reestablished his ability to form friendships with women and found this emotionally satisfying. He learned to enjoy the company of these female friends, and this encouraged him to think that he might be able to be "normal" after all. However, on the few occasions when he allowed any of these relationships to progress to sexual intimacy, he found himself fantasizing about men again. Heterosexual intimacy was just not satisfying. Even so, he continued to suppress any desire for homosexual interactions for fear of being caught and ridiculed by his peers. His conflict persisted.

During the summer that followed his first year of college, several events occurred that permanently changed the course of Roberto's life. The first of these was the final and total disintegration of the relationship between him and his parents—a relationship that, over the years, had swung between poor and neutral, but seldom much higher than that. The main problem had always been his mother. Mrs. V. was opinionated, outspoken, and loud. Her dominating maternal attentions left little room for independence or disagreements. But there were many disagreements, and these were heated and loud, especially as Roberto's adolescent years moved along. Their disagreements often became violent outbursts, with very unflattering epithets screamed at each other.

Mr. V., on the other hand, never really had been an active part of the problem. He rarely became involved in any of the arguments and seldom interfered with the details of his wife's management of the home. His concept of his "manly" role was to "make the important decisions" and to earn the living. Roberto and his father had little in common and therefore little to talk about. Mr. V. identified primarily with the Hispanic part of his ethnic heritage, including most of the manners and values of that subculture. Roberto's own ethnic heritage was more diluted because his mother was not Hispanic. Beyond that, he had come to feel that it was not necessary or appropriate to identify with any single ethnic group when they lived in such a cosmopolitan city. They agreed to disagree on this matter, as with most contemporary issues. But there was one issue that they could not resolve this way. The long postponed revelation of Roberto's secret to his parents never took place in a planned way. It eventually did happen, but by accident.

Roberto had become so unhappy living at home while going to college that he had been desperately trying to think of a way to live elsewhere. He could not afford to move into a dorm, and the idea of living in a men's dorm was somewhat frightening anyway, because it increased the possibility of being discovered. He also could not afford to rent his own apartment and continue with school at the same time. He finally decided that the only solution was to drop out of school for a while and go to work full time.

When he announced his decision, his mother's reaction was even more violent and vitriolic than he had anticipated. In the heated exchange of yelling and insults that ensued, Roberto unintentionally blurted out that the happiest consequence for him of his decision was that he would never again have to live with a bitch like her, since he would eventually be living with a man! For the first time in his memory, his mother was stunned into silence. However, the full implication of the statement was also not missed by his father, who could not help overhearing the argument. The emotional outburst from Mr. V. totally filled the silence left by his mother, who had collapsed into a chair from shock and disbelief. Roberto was told to be out of the house as soon as possible, and that there would be no more financial assistance. The shame and embarrassment of having a *joto* for a son was more than his father could tolerate. He could not stand to look at him anymore.

In a matter of days Roberto had moved into his own apartment. He increased his work hours to full time and applied for a leave of absence from school for the following year. He did not speak with either of his parents again for nearly two years.

While leaving home can be a somewhat frightening experience for a late teenager, the year that followed Roberto's departure was the most satisfying of his life to that point. He reveled in the freedom from rules and regulations. And, although the new freedom was accompanied by new responsibilities, these turned out to be no problem. He managed his money well and was able to buy personal material things without having to ask for money or assistance, and without being questioned about his decisions. He was able to choose new friends without restriction, and in general, had a comfortable and secure feeling of control over his life.

However, there continued to be that one area of discontent. His late-adolescent sexual urges were stronger than ever and his frustration was a persistent distraction. "But I continued to deny myself the option of having sex with a man, no matter how explicit my sexual fantasies became." Determined as he was to hold on to this conviction, his inhibition and resolve were finally weakened by two unpleasant experiences. The combination effect of these incidents persuaded him that it might be all right at least to try experiencing what he secretly had been desiring. The first incident happened on the eve of his twentieth birthday. He was seduced by an aggressive young woman. Although he had no interest in having sex with her, the situation rapidly got out of hand. He felt helpless to control what was happening, primarily because it put him into a difficult personal conflict. He felt that if he refused he would be "found out." On the other hand, he felt that if he went along and was unsuccessful, he also could be labeled as unmanly. He felt intense pressure to perform and perform well, but he had no desire to perform at all. He managed to fake his way through the trial, but resolved never again to allow himself to be trapped in a similar situation.

Not long after this experience, a good friend invited Roberto to participate in a three-way (a ménage à trois). Intrigued by the idea and flattered by the invitation, he agreed. Once again, he found himself in a difficult conflict. The fantasy was attractive, but the reality was repulsive. The experience was heterosexual and provided no outlet for his homosexual fantasies. He was further repulsed by what seemed like sexual competition with his friend. All in all, the experience was a miserable failure and, as he perceived it, damaging to his credibility as a heterosexual in the eyes of his friends. In fact, although they were aware of his frustration and impotence, there was no evidence that they understood why. Nevertheless, he was uneasy and self-conscious for several days.

The personal impact of these two experiences convinced Roberto that he had to make a significant change in his life-style. Attempting to live a lie in a heterosexual environment was frustrating and unpleasant, and was simply not working. Furthermore, he was tired of living with the constant pressure and anxiety of being discovered. Although he disliked the idea of leaving his friends, he decided that what he needed at this time was to spend time in an environment where homosexuality was accepted. He needed to be where he could be anonymous for a while, to decide what he really wanted and who he was. He gave notice to his employer, arranged to sublet his apartment, and took off for San Francisco.

In his fantasies, Roberto pictured San Francisco as a place where homosexual relationships could be quickly and easily arranged. He had read that in some areas homosexuality was the norm. And while he found both of these things to be true in the California city, he also encountered a few surprises as a result of his sexual and geographical naïveté. "What I had not anticipated was the transitory nature of most gay relationships there. Nor was I prepared for the paradoxical attitude of many homosexuals. They may desire and seek out a lasting relationship—but only if it does not interfere with the freedom to be sexually active with others, if they choose. Among many homosexuals, promiscuity is a way of life. On the other hand, I observed many homosexuals involved in lasting and loyal monogamous relationships."

Although Roberto found the promiscuity to be a surprising and morally objectionable part of some gay behavior, he also confessed that he enjoyed this part of gay life during his stay in San Francisco. "It was like a second puberty," he said. He was able to make up for his relative lack of sexual experience and learn more about people at the same time. "It was also satisfying and uplifting to my self-concept to have people find me attractive. In spite of the moral conflict, I was comfortable with myself for the first time. It was also wonderful finally to have a peer group with whom I could genuinely identify."

With important personal questions resolved, Roberto found himself, several months later, becoming impatient to resume the education that he had temporarily put on hold. He returned to his home city with a new confidence that he could have both homosexual and heterosexual friends who accepted him for what he was. During that last conversation in my office, he said, "I must admit that there are times when it feels a little strange and complicated to be a homosexual in a predominantly heterosexual college environment. But being gay is a relatively small part of my personality, and it is the rest of what I am that is important—and I am relatively well adjusted and comfortable now."

During his second year of college he developed a best-friend relationship with another male student, who was also gay. The other young man eventually moved into Roberto's apartment, to share expenses and needs for intimacy. This close relationship was also therapeutic for both men, as they spent many hours talking through their past conflicts and confusions. Roberto also was helped by several talking sessions with a counselor at the college counseling center. During that school year he also made new friends, both male and female, with whom he was comfortable.

As for his parents, they began to experience loneliness and guilt following Roberto's separation from the home and they eventually sought counseling assistance. As a result of a referral to a support group for families of homosexuals, they found new friends with whom they could share feelings and experiences. In time, Mrs. V. came to accept her son's independence and individuality, and Mr. V. came to accept Roberto's homosexuality without hostility or a sense of blame. During the Christmas holidays, after Roberto's return to college, his parents initiated a renewed contact with him. Gradually and cautiously they formed a new relationship. By the end of the college year, the family had established a more loving and supportive relationship than Roberto had known in many years.

The last time I saw Roberto, he was walking across the stage to receive his associate degree. I saw a confident and well-adjusted young man, stepping out to make his independent way in the world. His parents were a proud and excited part of the audience that day.

QUESTIONS FOR DISCUSSION

1. How do you feel when you see a person acting in what you consider to be a homosexual manner, for example, when you see two people of the same sex behaving affectionately toward each other?
2. Why do you think you feel that way?
3. By what name do you refer to homosexuals? Is it an insulting name? Do you know the origin of the name?
4. To the best of your knowledge, what is the attitude of your parents toward homosexuals? Is it similar to or different from your own?
5. To what extent does your religious background influence your attitude toward homosexuality?
6. How would you react, or how have you reacted, when a person of the same sex made affectionate or sexual overtures toward you? Is/was your reaction somewhat violent? If so, why?
7. How would you feel if you discovered that your brother or sister was a homosexual? Would you then behave differently toward him or her?
8. Do you think you could be a friend to Roberto?
9. When and why do you think Roberto became a homosexual?
10. Do you think his homosexuality could be "cured"? Do you think he should try to be "cured"? How do you think he would respond to this suggestion?

BIBLIOGRAPHY

This discussion of homosexuality has been, by necessity and intent, only a brief overview of the subject in order to introduce our case study. I encourage the reader to do more extensive and thorough reading about homosexuality so as to be better informed about a complicated and controversial subject. Your primary textbook probably has a good chapter on sexuality. There are also a number of excellent books in the library devoted exclusively to human sexuality. Three books in particular that I found to be especially authoritative, thorough, and helpful are:

Judd Marmor (ed.). *Homosexual Behavior—A Modern Reappraisal.* Basic Books, Inc., New York, 1980.

Masters, W. H.; Johnson, V. E.; Kolodny, R. C. *Masters and Johnson on Human Sexuality and Loving.* Chapter 14. Little, Brown & Co., Boston, 1986.

Kenneth Plummer (ed.). *The Making of the Modern Homosexual.* Barnes and Noble Books, Totowa, NJ, 1981.

Chapter
12

Depression
The Common Cold of Mental Illness

EMILY D.: WHAT'S THE POINT OF GOING ON?

Introduction

How long has it been since you had one of those awful down days? Were down in the dumps. Had the blues. One of those days when you can't see the forest for the trees; can't see the world clearly because of all the problems. Nothing goes right or turns out right. If you are a college student, that bad day probably wasn't very long ago, maybe even yesterday. Being a college student isn't easy, and most college students are quite familiar with depression. In spite of the popular image of carefree college days, serious students probably have as many days dominated by fatigue and sadness as happy, carefree ones. But is this the depression the mental health professionals refer to when they speak of *the* mental illness of the eighties, or "the common cold of psychopathology," as Martin Seligman termed it? Not really. Clinical depression is a great deal more involved than the blue-mood days that we are all familiar with.

DEFINITIONS AND FORMS

Question: Is there a formal system for organizing and classifying the various forms of depression? Yes, but depression occurs in such a baffling array of forms and patterns that it becomes difficult to fit them into neat diagnostic categories. No matter what classification system we use to differentiate the forms, some categories always overlap. Some of the most important differences between the forms of depression are primarily a matter of degree. These many forms and intensities occur along a broad continuum. At the milder end is the occasional sadness, disillusionment, and fatigue resulting from loss or disappointment that everyone experiences. It usually doesn't last very long, giving way to more positive moods as life circumstances change. This form is labeled *situational* depression. From the disorders in the middle or moderate range of the continuum on up to the most serious forms, we have *clinical* depression. Thus *situational* and *clinical* are the two broadest categories used to classify depression.

Clinical depression is classified by mental illness professionals as a mood disorder or affective disorder. It is defined as an unpleasant emotional state dominated by prolonged deep sadness and apathy. Seriously depressed people are notable also for a severely negative self-concept; a tendency to avoid other people; dramatic changes in sleeping, eating, and sexual need patterns; and a profound lethargy and inability to function properly or normally. Clinical depression can last for weeks, months, or even years. In the most extreme forms the mental functioning of depressives may be psychotic. Their profoundly negative perceptions of life events and their own self-worth may bear no relation to objective reality. Delusions and hallucinations commonly intrude into their thinking. Clinical depression is often divided into two subcategories, according to the most important *cause* or *etiology* of a particular illness: (1) *Reactive* depression is brought on by unhappy life events such as the death of a loved one, the loss of an important possession or relationship, or failure to achieve important personal goals. (2) *Biological* depression is caused primarily by abnormal brain chemistry, usually high or low levels of certain critical neurotransmitters.

Clinical depression is also divided into two additional categories distinguished by different *behavior* patterns: *Major depression* is a one-way symptom pattern, in which the person is always down and deeply depressed for extended periods of time; and *Bipolar disorder*, which used to be called manic-depressive psychosis, is a pattern in which the depressed periods are interrupted by episodes of the opposite extreme—frantic, disorganized periods of overstimulated mental and physical activity. Sometimes the manic phase of this disorder is the predominant one. Clearly this is a situation where the brain has great difficulty maintaining its own homeostasis.

In addition to all of these, there is one more form of depression that only recently has been identified and labeled. It is called *seasonal affective disorder* or (*S.A.D.*). It provides a diagnostic category for those people who become deeply depressed and immobilized in the winter. Most of us probably can identify somewhat with the difficulty in "getting up" for the holiday season because of the cold and gloomy weather in December, along with the very short days and the decrease in sunshine. We may also have unpleasant memories that depress our mood. There is an increase in natural deaths and suicides at this time of the year. Some people are so seriously affected that they become totally disabled. Once more, a variety of factors is suspected, as we discuss in the following section. On short days the decreased sunlight affects the body's natural clock and production of chemicals in the brain. People with a genetic predisposition to depression seem to have a much greater vulnerability to S.A.D.

CAUSES

The cause of any particular episode of depression, whether minor or major, is often a combination of three variables: First, there is apt to be one or more unpleasant life events. There may have been a serious loss—death, divorce, or separation involving a loved one, a friend, or the loss of a valuable possession. There may be stress or anxiety-producing situations such as academic or job pressures, difficult life and career decisions, or unwelcome changes in one's life situation. There may have been failures to meet expectations of one's own or those of other important people in our lives, such as parents, loved ones, teachers, coaches, or employers.

Second, the unpleasant experience of these events may be exaggerated by one's *psychological predispositions*. A person may have a low sense of self-esteem, personal worth, or competence. This can cause unreasonable, pessimistic expectations regarding one's ability to control what is happening in one's life. This sense of helplessness is a common ingredient in depression. One may also be disposed to perceiving the seriousness of a situation in an exaggerated way. Even the slightest setback may be viewed as another pending disaster.

The third factor is *biological vulnerability*. There is a tendency for depression to run in successive generations of the same family. This means that there is a genetic predisposition—abnormal levels of the chemicals in the brain that affect moods and emotions.

No doubt there will always be disagreement and debate over which of these variables comes first or is the most important. Perhaps it is another unsolvable "chicken and egg" question. But each side of the argument can present persuasive evidence for their position. Many depressed people do not have any history of depression in their families. And many people from depression-susceptible families do not become depressed without stressful life events and/or self-concept deficiencies. Once more we are caught on the horns of the heredity vs. environment dilemma.

SYMPTOMS AND CHARACTERISTICS

If there are important differences between everyday depression and more serious clinical depression, how does one know when a loved one or friend should be referred for professional help? As we have suggested, the differences are primarily a matter of degree, how long the depression lasts, and how seriously the brain chemistry is disrupted. Therefore, it might be useful to list in more detail the characteristics of clinical depression. As we do so, notice the frequent contradictions which contribute to the confusing nature of the illness.

Clinical depression's many manifestations make it a total body illness, a total person illness. It affects not only mood and emotions, but body, thoughts, and behavior. There is a deep and continuing sadness and despair, descending into chronic apathy. The depressive eventually doesn't seem to care about anything. He doesn't seem to be able to care about anything. He feels "empty." There is a consistent low state of all aspects of the self-concept. The person may feel overwhelmed by a sense of worthlessness, incompetence, impotence, powerlessness, and helplessness. There is a general tendency to put oneself down, to be self-critical, and focus on failure and everything negative —"I'm just no good." Guilt and self-blame are other common manifestations.

The body functions at a low level of activity. Movements are slow, and there is little or no energy, drive, or enthusiasm. There is no longer any interest or pleasure in normal activities, hobbies, even sex. Some people lose interest in eating and lose weight. Others overeat and gain weight. Still others lose interest in eating but, oddly, gain weight anyway. Sleeping patterns become abnormal. Some people sleep too much; others have difficulty sleeping for very long or have a general insomnia problem. These difficulties, along with restlessness and irritability, are symptoms of anxiety and sympathetic nervous system activity—which contradicts the otherwise depressed level of body activity. Anxiety also may be manifested in digestive disorders, headache, and other pains and discomforts.

The mind may become obsessed with thoughts of hopelessness, helplessness, and pessimism. Thoughts of giving up, death, or suicide are common. The person may even plan suicide attempts, but ironically may have difficulty mustering the energy or determination to carry out the plans. The mind may have difficulty concentrating on anything, making decisions, or remembering what was important a short time earlier. The person just can't get the motor going. Productive work is impossible. The total resistance of this illness to any force of will or self-help attempt gradually leads the person into total despair.

All of these mental and physical disabilities result in behavior which is slow, indecisive, and purposeless. The person comes to avoid people and social activities altogether. You might hear the person express it this way: "They cannot understand, and will probably make ignorant suggestions. So why risk more failure—or bother with them at all?"

HOW TO COUNTERACT DEPRESSION

Some Personal Mental Health Suggestions

1. *Socialize. Do things with people.* Select good friends and loved ones— people who care about you—and try to think of reasons to be with them, rather than reasons to avoid them. *Talk* with friends. Perhaps even a session or three with a professional counselor would be appropriate and helpful. Do your share. Don't expect other people to do all of the helping work. Remember, persistent negative attitudes, talk, and behavior are a drain on people's patience. It can turn people off to being around you if they have to listen to you complain all the time.

2. *Work on the negative thinking.* Try to look at depressing events more

objectively. Ask yourself, "Is it really the disaster it appears to be? Listen to others who suggest a less negative way to look at things. Do things to distract your mind from negative thinking: Read a light, interesting book. Go to a good movie. Watch something engrossing on television.

3. *Get out of your cave.* Go out and do something a little more active and physical that you enjoy. Go for a walk. Ride a bike. Play a sport with a friend. Do something different and interesting. Go to church.

4. *Lighten the load.* Reexamine your goals and priorities. Perhaps some are unrealistically high. Perhaps a C is more reachable than an A. Decrease the chances of failure. Don't demand so much of yourself. Who said you had to be perfect anyway? Perhaps some tasks on your list are not as urgent as you thought. Set them aside until later. Break down large tasks into smaller ones. Take one task at a time, and one day at a time. Do not blame yourself for things that you cannot control. Guilt is a heavy load, so don't carry unnecessary guilt. Be patient and forgiving with yourself. The process of getting well may be slower than you would like. But the negative feelings and the negative thinking will eventually respond to treatment.

Suggestions for the Helping Person

The roles of the helper are simple but important.

1. *Don't expect too much of yourself as helper.* Depression can be a difficult, stubborn disorder. You are not likely to bring about a "cure" quickly or on your own.

2. *Be supportive and patient.* Offer understanding, affection, caring, encouragement, and patience. Be a good listener, but be ready to point out what is a more realistic assessment of a situation. Occasionally try to phrase your good ideas in the form of questions. A question tends to get attention better than a statement of advice. Offer a hopeful attitude to counteract the depressive's sense of hopelessness.

3. *Invite* the depressed person to do things that are more active, fun, cheerful, and diverting. Be gently assertive about this. There may be some resistance.

4. *Find out how to get professional help.* If the depression has persisted for some time, it is probable that more professional help is needed— perhaps even medication. Start by referral to the counseling psychologists at school. It should be someone who can determine when or if a more intensive combination of clinical psychology and medical expertise is called for.

To illustrate what we have been discussing in the technical introduction, let us now go on to read about a case which you might find on any campus. We'll call it the case of Emily D.

The Case of Emily D.

Toward the end of October, just past the middle of Emily's first semester in college, she found herself alone in her room on a Friday night. She was in a mood of solitary reflection and was engrossed in a personal reassessment. Looking back, what did her life add up to? Where was it going? She concluded that her college career was a disaster, with no hope for recovery. It probably never should have been attempted in the first place. It wasn't Emily's idea. Going to school had been a low priority for her since before she started high school. It was her mother who had insisted. It had not been negotiable. For Emily it had been an avoidance–avoidance conflict: Stay at home and endure the constant bickering and hateful fighting with her mother, or go away to college with its hated studying, unknown demands, and unsympathetic strangers. It was a no-win situation, but she had had no choice anyway.

It wasn't that she hadn't made any effort at all. For a while she had tried, but everything was a miserable failure in her eyes. Everyone else seemed to have friends and to be having a good time. But people told her that she was spoiled and selfish, and that she was whiney and so pessimistic that she was a "drag" to be around. "Well," she thought, "if I am spoiled and selfish, I sure must come by it naturally." Her mother never stopped being spoiled and selfish. But that was only part of it. Mrs. D. was at times a very sick woman. Emily hardly could remember her mother ever smiling. The corners of her mouth seemed permanently turned down, and her moods were mercurial and irrational. She could be vicious and cruel with her screaming accusations and verbal abuse. Emily bore many emotional scars from these assaults. She also had heard the horror stories about her mother's fits of depression and paranoia during her pregnancy with Emily. The postpartum depression had been so severe and irrational that Mr. D. had stopped visiting the hospital until it was time to bring his wife and infant home. Emily could remember her mother staying in bed for days at a time, totally incapacitated by her depression. And she had dreadful memories of the two occasions when her mother had been rushed to the hospital following suicide attempts.

Emily's father was more stable, but almost too much so. He was very rational and controlled, but had little aptitude for interaction on an emotional level. He was almost totally wrapped up in his successful business affairs, and thus was able to provide Emily with every *thing* that she needed or desired. But there was little or no emotional relationship, and certainly very little love was openly expressed. Thus Emily was both spoiled and deprived.

When Emily was 13, her father finally left the uncomfortable home, and her parents were divorced. Less than two years later he was remarried to a younger woman, who liked to have a good time and was "fun to be with." Emily's prolonged exercise in self-pity probably dated more from this traumatic event than from any other point in her life. She stayed with her mother, but life in the home from then on became even more of a hell. Her mother's normally sour disposition turned into a chronic hateful bitterness and resentment of Emily's father and "his new whore." Mrs. D. always had been a fairly heavy drinker, but now she drank more heavily and regularly than before. In fact, she was at least semi-inebriated most of the time.

Mrs. D.'s divorce settlement was financially generous, and Emily was well provided for. But the happy moments in her life from this point on were rare and fleeting. She occasionally visited her father but usually felt she was an inconvenience and an intruder into the new relationship. Her stepmother had little interest or aptitude for assuming motherly responsibilities. Also, the differences in age and personality prevented their being friends.

By this time Emily's self-worth was consistently locked into a low setting. She was wrapped up in feelings of abandonment, desertion, and loss. It became a repeating habit pattern, almost an obsession. "Nobody cares about me; nobody cares what happens to me," "Poor me, poor me." She learned to manipulate her parents by being a demanding brat—"Appease me for neglecting me." And they complied. Buying her things was an easy way to compensate for being wrapped up in their own affairs.

Low self-worth has a very stupefying effect, so Emily felt virtually incapable of learning, and had no interest in even trying. She coasted through high school, and searched for purposeless activities and excitement to pass the time. She hung around with whatever group would accept her. Her money and ability to buy alcohol and drugs bought her some friends—even a few boyfriends—for short periods. But there were no close friendships, no intimacies.

At the end of the twelfth grade, Emily was one of a large group of students who were given high school diplomas—solely on the basis of an informal agreement between student and school system that they had "done their time." Emily was grateful that the obligation was over, even though she often had gone to school because it was better than being at home. A few weeks later she was shocked to discover that her mother was actively trying to enroll her in college for the following September. Emily had no intention of going along with this plan, so the summer was marked by frequent temper tantrums and tearful screaming arguments—all to no avail. On Labor Day she was packed off to an expensive private junior college—the only "decent" school that would accept her. Her mother had been very determined in this matter, especially since Emily's father had to pay for it.

Emily cried most of the time for the first couple of weeks. She was miserable and unhappy. College was a shock—every aspect of it. She didn't like not having her own room and her own bathroom. The girls she had to live with didn't let her have her own way all of the time, as she was used to. The food was horrible. In spite of a wide variety of choices in the college cafeteria, Emily decided that she didn't like any of it. She called both of her parents often, tearfully begging to come home. But neither parent would let her do so. The first semester was paid for and she was going to stay there. She was additionally "destroyed" to learn that she had been "replaced" in her mother's life by a new live-in boyfriend! He was young, a sometime actor, and her mother was supporting him. Emily was overwhelmed by feelings of being abandoned, cast out, unwanted, and unloved. She was bitter and angry and wanted to smash out at the whole world. She was finally referred to the college counseling center by a sympathetic dormitory resident director. The center was well prepared for the anticipated cases of first month home-sickness.

With the assistance of a counselor, Emily came to realize that sitting around feeling sorry for herself really solved none of her problems. She also came to accept that she had few options but to try to make the best of the situation. Perhaps she could learn to make a new life for herself. Unfortunate-ly, the fact remained that Emily was very poorly equipped to make the most of it. She had no training or aptitude for being empathic to other people's needs. Her roommates had developed such an attitude of intolerance for her selfish-ness and self-pity that they tended to just ignore her. As a result, they didn't even recognize her first fumbling efforts to be sociable or cooperative. The same was somewhat true of her other college acquaintances.

When she resolved to pay some serious attention to the neglected re-quirements of her courses of study, Emily was in for a worse shock. College in-structors actually expected her to do most of the work. This required many hours of study every week. At that point in the semester she was already far behind in required work and had failed nearly all of the tests that she had taken. When she really tried to study, most of the material made no sense to her at all. She had very elementary verbal skills and virtually no study skills. She had had no organized practice in how to correctly use the English language since the fifth or sixth grade, and her vocabulary never advanced beyond that level. Since a minimal level of math competency was required, she was enrolled in a freshman remedial math course. Even here she was helpless. She hated math.

As the days and weeks went by, life for Emily became a predictable se-quence of attempt and failure, leading to disappointment, decreased self-confidence, anxiety, depression. As self-pity and negative thinking began to intrude again, Emily reverted to habit patterns formed in high school and, following the lead of a number of other students in her dorm, she sought some diversion. She started going to drinking and drug parties, even during the week. This impulsive and very nonintegrative behavior not only consumed what could have been valuable study time, but left her in worse condition for class the next day. It also introduced another complication—she started try-ing to buy attention, acceptance, and affection by getting involved in a series of sexually promiscuous affairs with young men whom she met at parties. The affairs were always short term and followed the same pattern. Her partners would take advantage of her availability, use her, and then abandon her. Each affair was followed by dejection, and then worry and anxiety that she might be pregnant or have caught some disease. This provided another reason for self-deprecation.

By the middle of November there was ample empirical evidence to rein-force Emily's natural pessimism and her growing attitude of, "What's the use of trying anyway?" There had been nothing but try again, failure, disappoint-ment, and guilt. Her depression returned in earnest. An overwhelming lethargy replaced her former resolve. She couldn't make herself get up for classes. She responded to none of her roommate's admonitions. She was obsessed with thoughts of being worthless and helpless. In her distorted perception, she had no home, no friends, no love, no purpose, no resources. Her mood was dominated by hopelessness, futility, and emptiness. Her sleep became troubled and irregular. She became ill with a cold and was miserable with various aches and pains. She lost all interest in eating, or any other kind of self-care. But, for some reason she gained weight anyway and became quite overweight. Her appearance became sloppy and unkempt. There was the paradox of her expensive clothes and jewelry being worn in the most slovenly manner. After a while she settled into wearing nothing but the same dirty, wrinkled sweatsuit.

When strongly urged to return to talk with her counselor, she did so with reluctance and total lack of enthusiasm. The counseling sessions were very difficult. Emily did not want to talk and gave the impression that it was difficult even to summon the energy to do so. What did emerge were incomplete utterances that seemed to come from the depths of a dark pit. It was an interrupted stream of complaints, self-pity, overdefensiveness, projection, paranoia, and despair: "All of the girls are snobs, ... all of the boys are creeps, ... all of the teachers are unfair, ... the world stinks, ... you don't really care, ... nobody cares, ... nobody understands." All of this would be interspersed with vulgar, crude expletives, but with no emotional arousal to drive them. In fact, her words were barely audible. It was difficult, even for the experienced counselor, to remain objective and not have negative feelings in this situation.

The last straw came about a week before Thanksgiving. Emily called both her parents to find out which home she would be going to for the holiday. Each parent told her to spend the weekend with the other, because both couples were going away on vacation. When Emily complained that all of the school facilities would be shut down for the holiday, including the cafeteria, her mother told her, "All right, you can stay here if you want to be by yourself."

Emily's roommates became frightened by her talk of suicide later that week and alerted the dormitory resident director. She, in turn, discussed the situation with the director of the counseling center once more. Emily's counselor became quite concerned, because of a previous incident when Emily had nearly overdosed on a combination of drugs. At the time they had been unable to judge whether the overdose had been accidental or intentional. There had been some evidence that the incident was a cry for attention and help. The college's psychiatric consultant was called into the case, and Emily was brought to the infirmary for observation and supervision. The following day, the psychiatrist called Emily's father, recommending that she be brought home for supervised psychiatric treatment. (Emily's mother suddenly had gone into another severe depressive episode of her own, and was in no condition to be of any assistance in the matter.) That weekend, her father brought Emily home for good. Her college career was an unrecoverable failure.

QUESTIONS FOR DISCUSSION

1. Think of the continuum of severity of depression, described early in the chapter. Where do you think Emily's case ought to be placed along this continuum—at various times in her story?
2. Do you tend to feel optimistic or pessimistic about the long-range outcome of Emily's story? What are the reasons for your view?
3. Do you now better understand the complicated interrelationship between heredity and environment in the occurrence of depression? Do you have an opinion about which is the more influential cause of most cases of depression?
4. Do you know anyone like Emily? Do you feel you now are better able to intercede or be helpful?
5. Do you feel disposed to blame anyone for Emily's condition? Who? Why?
6. How much do you think that the nature of Emily's self-concept contributed to her maladjustment?

Appendix
Some Important Terms and Concepts

In Chapter 1, we devoted some considerable space and attention to the controversial and long-debated question(s) of what are the most important and valid criteria to use when judging whether a particular adjustive behavior or a general adjustive pattern results in a good healthy adjustment or a poorly adjusted condition. Chapter 1 also urged the student to discard the popular but technically useless terms "normal" and "abnormal" when trying to convey the idea of well adjusted or badly adjusted, in either everyday or technical conversation. At the time I suggested that we should instead substitute the terms *integrative* and *nonintegrative* for this purpose. These are terms which I have personally found useful in my teaching experience. To assure that the student will have a thorough understanding of these terms, I would like to give a more complete explanation of the terms here.

The concepts of integrative and nonintegrative are taken from a book which I used in the early years of my teaching, *The Psychology of Adjustment*, by Shaffer and Shoben.* It was an excellent textbook and I was disappointed when it went out of print some years ago. I have always been surprised that the words integrative and nonintegrative did not appear in more general usage in psychology, since they come closer to representing absolute criteria for evaluating the quality of adjustment than any other terms that I know of.

But before I discuss these terms, let me clarify some other basic language first. A frequent frustration to this teacher is the inconsistent use of the verb to adjust in psychology of adjustment textbooks. For example, using the word

---

*Shaffer, L. F., and Shoben, E. J., Jr. *The Psychology of Adjustment* (2nd ed.). Boston: Houghton Mifflin, 1956.

adjusted to mean well adjusted. This can be inaccurate and confusing to the student. The opposite of adjusted is not admusted; whereas some authors use adjusted and maladjusted as opposites. Correctly, well adjusted and maladjusted are opposites. A person who is adjusted to his anxieties or other tensions may in fact be a very unhealthy personality, psychologically speaking (and possibly physically unhealthy). Alcoholics and other drug addicts, compulsives, phobics, and other neurotics may quite successfully (though temporarily) control their anxieties and other tensions through the use of psychoactive drugs or defense mechanisms. However, from an overall point of view, they may be very sick people indeed. Therefore, we must use the word adjusted only as a neutral term without any implication of good or bad. Adjustment can mean only *tension reduction*. Adjusted can only mean tensions are reduced. To speak of being well adjusted or poorly adjusted we must use modifying terms. In short, we need some language which will enable us to communicate clearly to each other the idea of healthy adjustment or unhealthy adjustment.

This brings us to the terms *integrative* and *nonintegrative* to solve our semantic problem. If we look up the word *integrate* in the dictionary, we find that it means to make whole by bringing all parts together. The related word, integral, means essential for completion, an important constituent part. Therefore, an integrative adjustment is one that takes into consideration all of a person's needs. It does not take care of just one need while slighting or ignoring others. An integrative adjustment is also integrative with respect to time. It does not focus exclusively on present tensions while ignoring or making more difficult future adjustments. An integrative adjustment also takes into consideration that a person needs to maintain an accepted place in social groups—so it does not interfere with other people's needs or their rights. Out of the many choices available in an adjustive situation, an integrative adjustment considers long-term goals as well as immediate needs.

On the other hand, a nonintegrative behavior or adjustment is the opposite of all these characteristics. It is maladjustive because it only is concerned with reducing immediate tensions immediately, by whatever means are at hand. It ignores long-term consequences and other important needs as well as other people's needs. It never considers postponing immediate gratification for the sake of overall and long-term healthy adjustment. It is literally not well integrated into a person's total pattern of needs, including having an accepted and respected place in society.

The terms are easy to illustrate with a familiar example. Take the case of Joe, a first-year college student. Adjusting to the new environment, the new independence, and the new demands and challenges is a formidable task for almost all young people who attempt it. And they bring with them several strong patterns of motivation. Certainly two of the most important of these are academic motivation and social motivation. Every student needs to achieve good grades in order to maximize his or her options after college and to grow as a person in a social context. Let's say that as the freshman year progresses Joe is encountering some serious problems with the first of these. His grades in his college courses are unacceptably low and he is experiencing a lot of tension from the pressures coming from his parents, the dean's office, and his own frustration. There are many choices available for dealing with this problem and the tensions it produces. Joe could talk with his instructors for advice and counsel on how he might improve his grades in each course. He could seek assistance to improve his study habits and to learn to organize his time better. He could do extra credit projects in some of his courses. He could talk with other students who are having better success, or avail himself of the peer tutors. He might seek help at the counseling center to explore the possibility of having chosen the wrong major or that there might be personal problems interfering with his concentration. If any combination of these activities results in better academic success, then he will have reduced his tension while solving the *underlying problem* at the same time. Furthermore, if his academic work becomes more efficient he might enjoy more tension-free time to develop comfortable social relationships or organized group activities, and with an improved sense of self-esteem or less of a sense of failure. These adjustive choices can be described as integrative because they are integrated into the person's total pattern of needs, present and future, including social acceptance, because they do not violate other people's needs and rights, and because they deal with the problem as well as the tension.

In contrast, Joe could choose from the many other adjustment options which are popular among college students. The number of widely proclaimed rationalizations is limitless: "All the other students are cheating, I can't compete with that." "It's the instructor's fault, I can't understand what he is saying." "The instructor doesn't like me, I couldn't pass his course no matter what I did." "I've been sick." "The college food gives me indigestion." "I'm a night person, I can't function in the daytime." "They don't make the courses interesting; I'm too bored to study that stuff." Joe could try cheating on the tests and papers himself—at the risk of automatically failing the course if he is caught. He could find reasons not to take tests, relieving his pretest anxiety, but somehow ignoring the fact that this will result in a 0 for a test score in the instructor's grade book. He could brag about how much smarter he is than his grades show. He could start drinking heavily and using other psychoactive drugs to relieve his anxiety, and help him pretend that no problem exists. He might increasingly resort to the substitution of daydreams for real satisfactions. Such behaviors would probably reduce his tensions, and are therefore adjustive behaviors. However, they are nonintegrative adjustments because they are only temporary, because they do not solve the problem or even attempt to deal with it, because they make future adjustments even more difficult, and because they ignore or violate other people's rights.

There are many other common examples of nonintegrative adjustments from real-life behavior. A person might displace the anger and aggression from his frustration by hitting out at other, weaker persons or by smashing things—and thus get into more trouble. There are millions of people who maintain a tension reduction through the use of alcohol and other drugs, while they are destroying their brains and ruining and shortening their lives.

This is probably the best and simplest example of nonintegrative behavior. There also are millions of young people who numb their brains and senses and drown out the world by listening to loud musical noise. This sedation is achieved at the cost of permanent loss of sensitivity of their hearing (not to mention the alienation of other people around them whose ears have not lost their sensory acuity). There are some who would say that our present culture is rampant with nonintegrative, self-destructive behaviors, resulting from the demand for immediate gratification and lack of caution and foresight for consequences. The trend toward uninhibited sexuality, for example, has resulted in an epidemic of irreversible diseases such as AIDS and herpes and of unwanted pregnancies. On a simpler level, when one gorges on unripe fruit or candy or alcohol to immediately satisfy one's hunger or thirst, then one pays the price later in the form of a stomach ache, or diarrhea, or fat, or an awful hangover.

There is a third quantity of adjustment, which is not on the integrative–nonintegrative continuum. It may be called *nonadjustment*. This term refers to behaviors that are responses to problems and tension, but do not have any tension-reducing value. A typical nonadjustive response would be simply restless pacing with worrying and fretting, and possibly wallowing in a continuous self-pity party. "Oh woe is me. I don't know what to do. Why does everything happen to me?"

An honest and objective examination of our own adjustive behaviors is likely to find examples of all three of these kinds of responses to problem tensions. The quality of one's adjustment is measured by the relative proportion of the three kinds of adjustments in one's behavior. A person whose adjustments are mostly integrative is likely to be a well-adjusted person. Neurotic behavior is almost by definition predominantly nonintegrative. A person who exhibits frequent nonadjustive behavior is also by definition poorly adjusted, and also is likely to manifest a variety of psychosomatic symptoms.

To paraphrase the nice summary statement at the end of the Shaffer and Shoben discussion: When you can satisfy your motives and needs without inappropriate emphasis on any one need or the slighting of other needs, and when you can do this with consideration for the adjustment needs of other people, then you are a well-adjusted person.